ClearRevise®

OCR GCSE
Physical Education J857

Illustrated revision and practice

Published by
PG Online Limited
The Old Coach House
35 Main Road
Tolpuddle
Dorset
DT2 7EW
United Kingdom

sales@pgonline.co.uk
www.clearrevise.com
www.pgonline.co.uk
2023

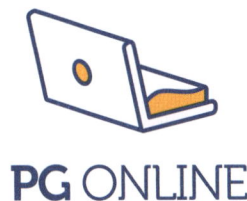

PREFACE

Absolute clarity! That's the aim.

This is everything you need to ace the exams and beam with pride. Each topic is laid out in a beautifully illustrated format that is clear, approachable and as concise and simple as possible.

Each section of the specification is clearly indicated to help you cross-reference your revision. The checklist on the contents pages will help you keep track of what you have already worked through and what's left before the big day.

We have included worked exam-style questions with answers. There is also a set of exam-style questions at the end of each section for you to practise writing answers. You can check your answers against those given at the end of the book.

LEVELS OF LEARNING

Based on the degree to which you are able to truly understand a new topic, we recommend that you work in stages. Start by reading a short explanation of something, then try to recall what you've just read. This will have a limited effect if you stop there but it aids the next stage. Question everything. Write down your own summary and then complete and mark a related exam-style question. Cover up the answers if necessary but learn from them once you've seen them. Lastly, teach someone else. Explain the topic in a way that they can understand. Have a go at the different practice questions – they offer an insight into how and where marks are awarded.

Design and artwork: Jessica Webb / PG Online Ltd

First edition 2023   10 9 8 7 6 5 4 3 2 1
A catalogue entry for this book is available from the British Library
ISBN: 978-1-916518-06-3
Copyright © PG Online 2023
All rights reserved
No part of this publication may be reproduced, stored in a retrieval system, or transmitted in any form or by any means without the prior written permission of the copyright owner.

Printed on FSC® certified paper by Bell and Bain Ltd, Glasgow, UK.

THE SCIENCE OF REVISION

Illustrations and words

Research has shown that revising with words and pictures doubles the quality of responses by students.[1] This is known as 'dual-coding' because it provides two ways of fetching the information from our brain. The improvement in responses is particularly apparent in students when they are asked to apply their knowledge to different problems. Recall, application and judgement are all specifically and carefully assessed in public examination questions.

Retrieval of information

Retrieval practice encourages students to come up with answers to questions.[2] The closer the question is to one you might see in a real examination, the better. Also, the closer the environment in which a student revises is to the 'examination environment', the better. Students who had a test 2–7 days away did 30% better using retrieval practice than students who simply read, or repeatedly reread material. Students who were expected to teach the content to someone else after their revision period did better still.[3] What was found to be most interesting in other studies is that students using retrieval methods and testing for revision were also more resilient to the introduction of stress.[4]

Ebbinghaus' forgetting curve and spaced learning

Ebbinghaus' 140-year-old study examined the rate at which we forget things over time. The findings still hold true. However, the act of forgetting facts and techniques and relearning them is what cements them into the brain.[5] Spacing out revision is more effective than cramming – we know that, but students should also know that the space between revisiting material should vary depending on how far away the examination is. A cyclical approach is required. An examination 12 months away necessitates revisiting covered material about once a month. A test in 30 days should have topics revisited every 3 days – intervals of roughly a tenth of the time available.[6]

Summary

Students: the more tests and past questions you do, in an environment as close to examination conditions as possible, the better you are likely to perform on the day. If you prefer to listen to music while you revise, tunes without lyrics will be far less detrimental to your memory and retention. Silence is most effective.[5] If you choose to study with friends, choose carefully – effort is contagious.[7]

---

1. Mayer, R. F. & Anderson, R. B. (1991). Animations need narrations: An experimental test of dual-coding hypothesis. *Journal of Education Psychology*, (83)4, 484–490.
2. Roediger III, H. L., & Karpicke, J.D. (2006). Test-enhanced learning: Taking memory tests improves long-term retention. *Psychological Science*, 17(3), 249–255.
3. Nestojko, J., Bui, D., Kornell, N. & Bjork, E. (2014). Expecting to teach enhances learning and organisation of knowledge in free recall of text passages. *Memory and Cognition*, 42(7), 1038–1048.
4. Smith, A. M., Floerke, V. A., & Thomas, A. K. (2016) Retrieval practice protects memory against acute stress. *Science*, 354(6315), 1046–1048.
5. Perham, N., & Currie, H. (2014). Does listening to preferred music improve comprehension performance? *Applied Cognitive Psychology*, 28(2), 279–284.
6. Cepeda, N. J., Vul, E., Rohrer, D., Wixted, J. T. & Pashler, H. (2008). Spacing effects in learning a temporal ridgeline of optimal retention. *Psychological Science*, 19(11), 1095–1102.
7. Busch, B. & Watson, E. (2019), *The Science of Learning*, 1st ed. Routledge.

CONTENTS

Paper 1 Physical factors affecting performance
Topic 1.1 Applied anatomy and physiology

Specification point ☑

1.1.a	Location of major bones	2 ☐
1.1.a	Functions of the skeleton	4 ☐
1.1.a	Types of synovial joint	5 ☐
1.1.a	Types of movement at hinge joints and ball and socket joints	6 ☐
1.1.b	Location of major muscle groups	8 ☐
1.1.b	The roles of muscle in movement	9 ☐
1.1.c	Lever systems	10 ☐
1.1.c	Mechanical advantage	12 ☐
1.1.c	Planes of movement and axes of rotation	13 ☐
1.1.d	Structure of the heart	14 ☐
1.1.d	Blood vessels	16 ☐
1.1.d	Heart rate, stroke volume and cardiac output	17 ☐
1.1.d	Structure and function of the respiratory system	18 ☐
1.1.d	Breathing rate and tidal volume	20 ☐
1.1.d	Aerobic and anaerobic exercise	21 ☐
1.1.e	The short-term effects of exercise	22 ☐
1.1.e	The long-term effects of exercise	24 ☐
	Examination practice 1.1	26 ☐

Topic 1.2 Physical training

Specification point ☑

1.2.a	The components of fitness	29 ☐
1.2.b	The principles of training	37 ☐
1.2.b	Types of training	38 ☐
1.2.b	Interval training	40 ☐
1.2.b	The key components of a warm up	43 ☐
1.2.b	The key components of a cool down	44 ☐
1.2.c	Preventing injury in physical activity and training	45 ☐
1.2.c	Hazards in sport settings	46 ☐
	Examination practice 1.2	47 ☐

Paper 2   Socio-cultural issues and sports psychology

Topic 2.1   Socio-cultural influences

Specification point ☑

2.1.a	Physical activity and sport in the UK	50 ☐
2.1.a	Factors affecting participation in physical activity and sport	51 ☐
2.1.a	Strategies to improve participation	55 ☐
2.1.b	Commercialisation of sport	56 ☐
2.1.b	Types of media	57 ☐
2.1.b	Sponsorship and the media	58 ☐
2.1.c	Ethics in sport	60 ☐
2.1.c	Violence in sport	61 ☐
2.1.c	Drugs in sport	62 ☐
	Examination practice 2.1	64 ☐

Topic 2.2   Sports psychology

Specification point ☑

2.2	Characteristics of skilful movement	66 ☐
2.2	Classification of skills	67 ☐
2.2	Goal setting	68 ☐
2.2	Mental preparation	69 ☐
2.2	Types of guidance	70 ☐
2.2	Types of feedback	72 ☐
	Examination practice 2.2	73 ☐

Topic 2.3   Health, fitness and well-being

Specification point ☑

2.3	Health, fitness and well-being	75 ☐
2.3	The health benefits of physical activity	76 ☐
2.3	The consequences of a sedentary lifestyle	77 ☐
2.3	Balanced diet	78 ☐
2.3	Nutrition	79 ☐
2.3	Effect of hydration on energy use	80 ☐
	Examination practice 2.3	81 ☐

The use of data

Understanding how data is collected	84
Presenting data	85
Analysis and evaluation of data	86
Examination practice	**88**

Non-exam assessment (NEA)

Practical performances	90
Analysis and evaluation or performance	91

Examination practice answers	**92**
Levels-based mark schemes for extended response questions	99
Index	100
Examination tips	**105**

MARK ALLOCATIONS

Green mark allocations[1] on answers to in-text questions throughout this guide help to indicate where marks are gained within the answers. A bracketed '1' e.g. [1] = one valid point worthy of a mark. In longer answer questions, a mark is given based on the whole response. In these answers, a judgement should be made using the levels-based mark scheme on page 99. There are often many more points to make than there are marks available so you have more opportunity to max out your answers than you may think.

TOPICS FOR PAPER 1
Physical factors affecting performance (J587/01)

Information about Component 1

Mandatory written exam: 1 hour
60 marks
30% of the qualification grade
Externally assessed.
All questions are mandatory.
Use black ink. You can use an HB pencil, but only for graphs and diagrams.
Calculators are permitted in this examination.

Specification coverage
1.1 Applied anatomy and physiology
1.2 Physical training

Questions
This paper consists of a mixture of objective response and multiple-choice questions, short answers and extended response items.
The use of data analysis skills are spread across all components and topics throughout the course.

LOCATION OF MAJOR BONES

The structure and function of the musculoskeletal system depends on the location of major bones and joints within the skeleton.

Bones in the human body

Cranium

The **cranium** comprises the facial bones and those that protect the brain, to form the **head**.

Humerus

The **humerus** is the upper arm bone, between the elbow and the scapula at the shoulder.

Vertebrae

The cranium is attached to the **spine**, which is usually made up of up to 33 **vertebrae**. The vertebrae protect the spinal cord.

Tarsals and metatarsals

The **tarsals** are located in the **ankle** and connect the **metatarsal** bones to the foot, in a similar way that the metacarpals do for the hand. **Metatarsals** are the bones inside the foot that connect to the toes (phalanges).

Ribs

The chest contains 12 **ribs** on each side, ten of which are connected to the **sternum** (the breast plate) to form a protective cage around your vital inner organs and aid respiration.

Pelvis

The **pelvis** comprises two parts that connect the upper body to the legs.

Femur

The **femur** is the upper leg bone and the largest in the human body.

A downhill skier has fallen with a suspected fracture of the lower leg, above the ankle. Name **one** of the bones that they may have fractured. [1]

Tibia,[1] *or fibula.*[1]

Infants are born with about 270 bones in their skeleton to provide extra flexibility. During childhood, many bones fuse together ending up with typically 210 bones in the adult skeleton.

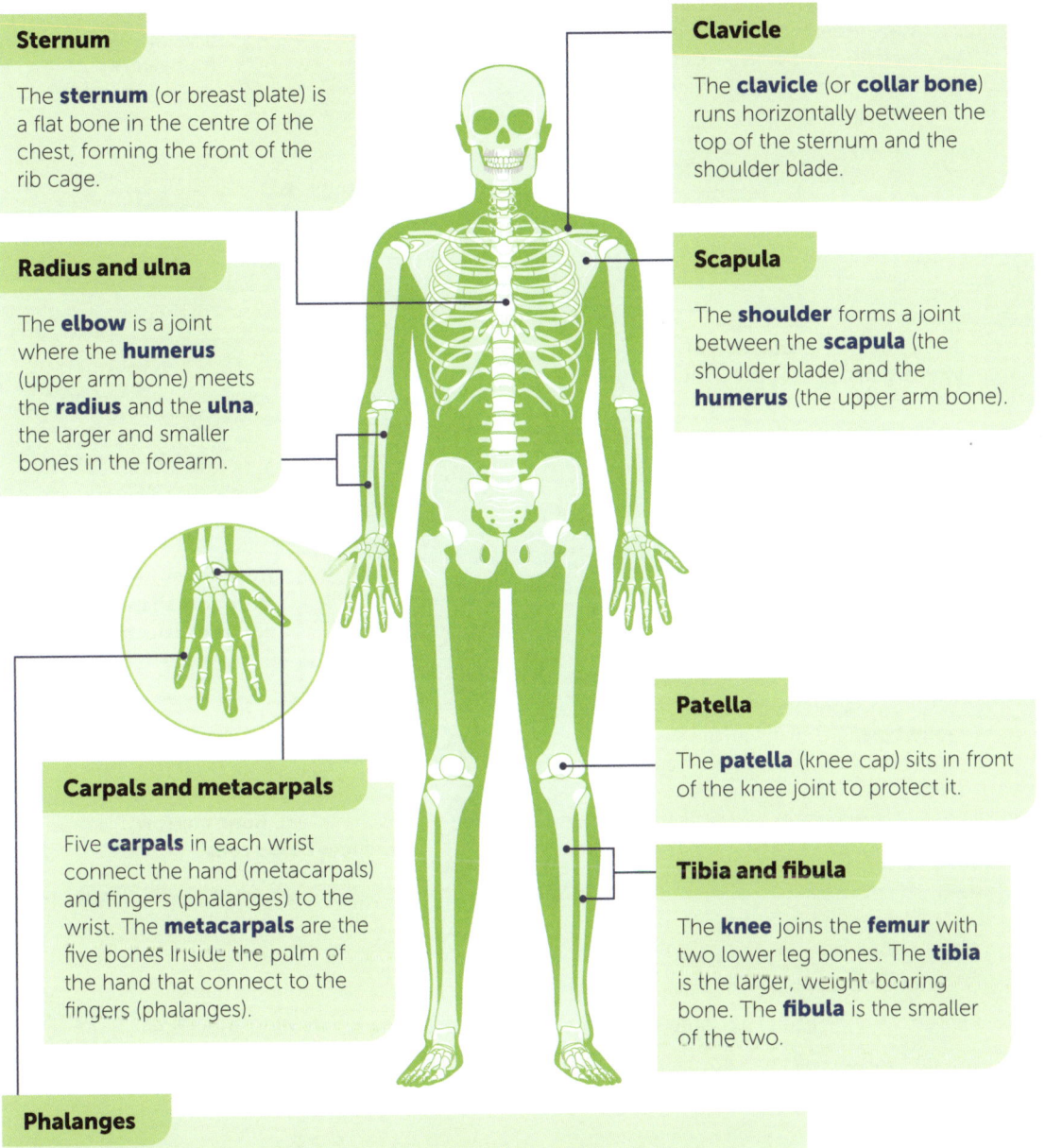

Sternum

The **sternum** (or breast plate) is a flat bone in the centre of the chest, forming the front of the rib cage.

Radius and ulna

The **elbow** is a joint where the **humerus** (upper arm bone) meets the **radius** and the **ulna**, the larger and smaller bones in the forearm.

Carpals and metacarpals

Five **carpals** in each wrist connect the hand (metacarpals) and fingers (phalanges) to the wrist. The **metacarpals** are the five bones inside the palm of the hand that connect to the fingers (phalanges).

Clavicle

The **clavicle** (or **collar bone**) runs horizontally between the top of the sternum and the shoulder blade.

Scapula

The **shoulder** forms a joint between the **scapula** (the shoulder blade) and the **humerus** (the upper arm bone).

Patella

The **patella** (knee cap) sits in front of the knee joint to protect it.

Tibia and fibula

The **knee** joins the **femur** with two lower leg bones. The **tibia** is the larger, weight-bearing bone. The **fibula** is the smaller of the two.

Phalanges

The **phalanges** are a group of 14 bones in each hand. Three in each of the **fingers** and two in the thumb. They are also found in the **toes** of each foot.

OCR GCSE **Physical Education** – Topic 1.1

1.1.a

FUNCTIONS OF THE SKELETON

The skeletal system provides a framework for movement. The muscular system attaches to the skeleton. When muscles contract, they pull the bones.

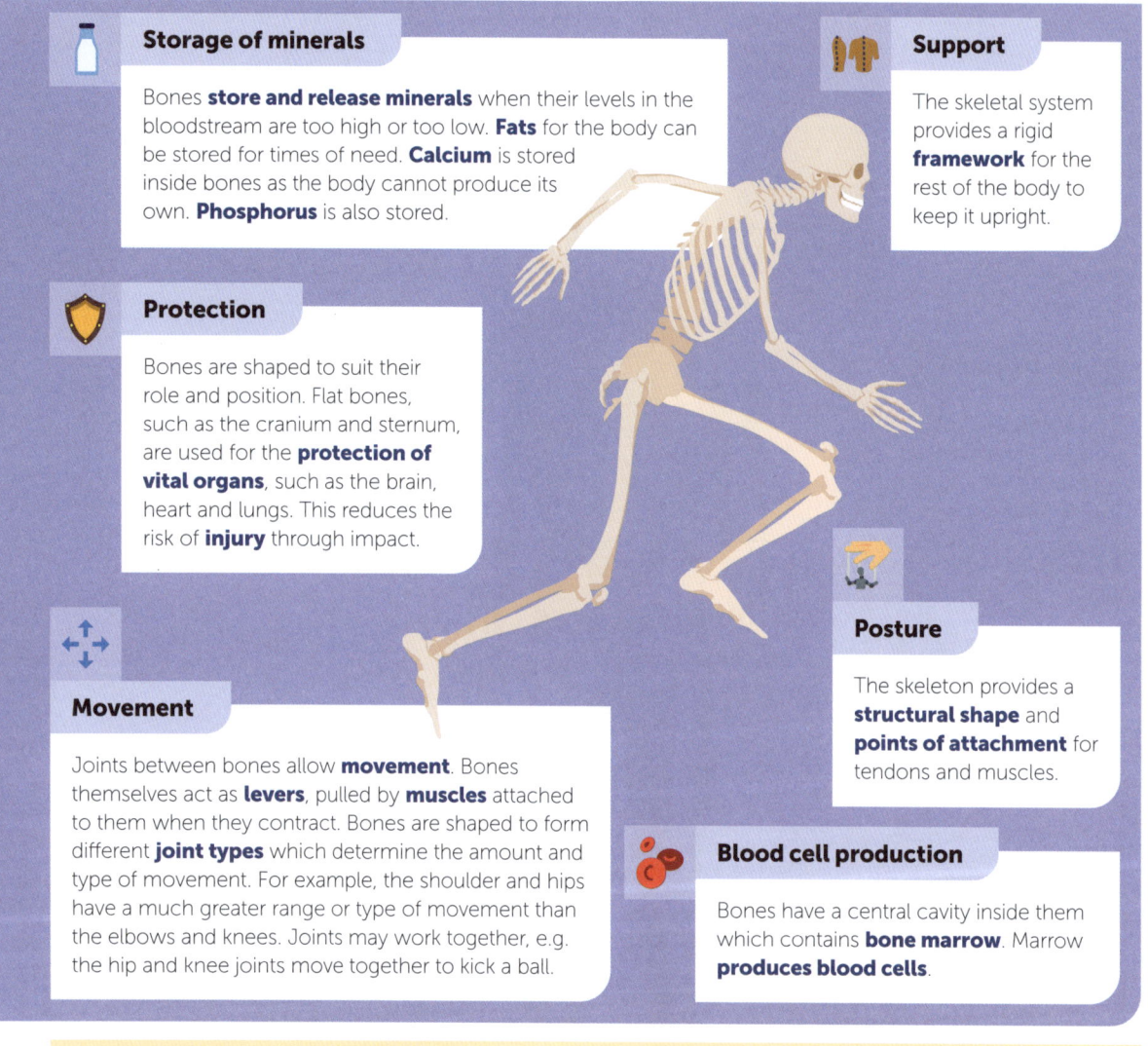

Storage of minerals

Bones **store and release minerals** when their levels in the bloodstream are too high or too low. **Fats** for the body can be stored for times of need. **Calcium** is stored inside bones as the body cannot produce its own. **Phosphorus** is also stored.

Support

The skeletal system provides a rigid **framework** for the rest of the body to keep it upright.

Protection

Bones are shaped to suit their role and position. Flat bones, such as the cranium and sternum, are used for the **protection of vital organs**, such as the brain, heart and lungs. This reduces the risk of **injury** through impact.

Movement

Joints between bones allow **movement**. Bones themselves act as **levers**, pulled by **muscles** attached to them when they contract. Bones are shaped to form different **joint types** which determine the amount and type of movement. For example, the shoulder and hips have a much greater range or type of movement than the elbows and knees. Joints may work together, e.g. the hip and knee joints move together to kick a ball.

Posture

The skeleton provides a **structural shape** and **points of attachment** for tendons and muscles.

Blood cell production

Bones have a central cavity inside them which contains **bone marrow**. Marrow **produces blood cells**.

Maya plays rugby.
  (a) Describe **one** way in which Maya's skeleton protects her vital organs during a game. [1]
  (b) Explain, with the use of a related sporting example, how Maya's bones allow movement. [2]

  (a) Her ribs will protect her heart and lungs in a scrum or tackle.[1] Her skull will help to protect her brain in a tackle.[1] Her sternum will protect her chest in a tackle.[1]
  (b) The femur acts as a lever[1] to generate speed when running to gain ground.[1] Muscles attached to bones pull the ulna/radius/femur to impart a force / range of motion on the ball when kicking / passing.[1] This allows Maya to pass more quickly / take longer penalties to benefit gameplay.[1]

TYPES OF SYNOVIAL JOINT

A synovial joint connects two or more bones within a joint capsule, allowing a wide range of movement to occur.

Structure of a synovial joint (the knee)

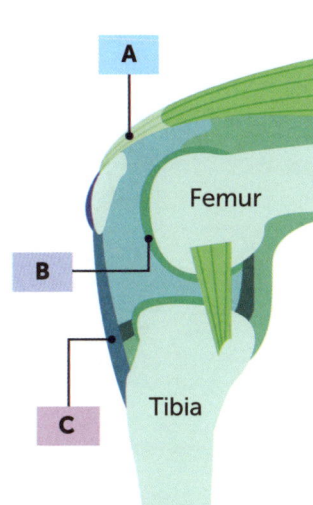

Femur
Tibia

A Tendons
Tendons are a tough yet flexible band of fibrous tissue which join muscles to bones, pulling them when muscles contract.

B Cartilage
Cartilage is a tough, elastic, fibrous connective tissue. It absorbs shock and acts as a cushion between the bones. It prevents bones from rubbing together directly, reducing wear and friction.

C Ligaments
Ligaments are short bands of tough and flexible tissue connecting bones together and stabilising a joint to prevent dislocation. Elasticity in the ligaments absorbs shock.

Joints

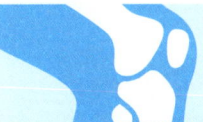

Hinge joints
The **elbows** and **knees** are example of hinge joints. They allow movement in one plane through flexion and extension with up to 180 degrees of motion.

Elbow – Articulating bones: humerus, radius, ulna.
Knee – Articulating bones: femur, tibia.

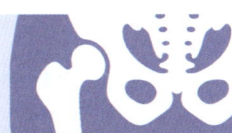

Ball and socket joints
The **shoulders** and **hips** are examples of ball and socket joints. A ball-shaped end of one bone fits into a cup-shaped socket in another. This allows for flexion and extension, abduction and adduction, circumduction and rotational movement in almost all directions, making sporting actions such as a cricket bowl or breaststroke swimming possible.

Shoulder – Articulating bones: humerus, scapula.
Hip – Articulating bones: pelvis, femur.

David is a competitive rock climber. His shoulders, elbows and knees are in constant use.
Describe the role of cartilage and ligaments in the prevention of injury. [3]

Cartilage absorbs shock[1] / provides a buffer between bones, preventing direct friction[1] / aids mobility or movement.[1]
Ligaments provide elasticity to absorb shock[1] / help keep the joint together by connecting bone to bone[1] / provide stability or restrict movement.[1]

TYPES OF MOVEMENT AT HINGE JOINTS AND BALL AND SOCKET JOINTS

The following types of movement are linked to specific types of joint, which enable that movement to take place.

Hinge joints

Flexion and extension

Flexion and **extension** occurs at hinge joints such the **elbows** and **knees**, as the angle of the joint closes and opens.

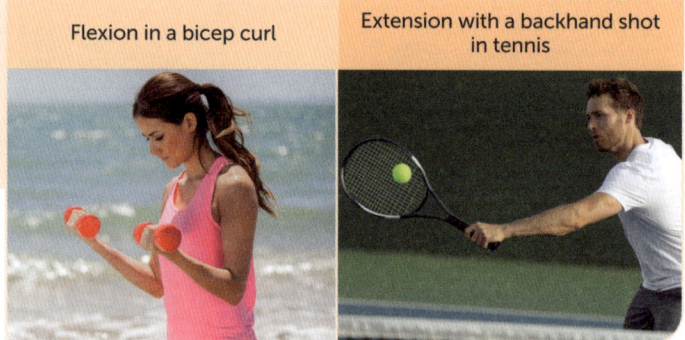

Flexion in a bicep curl

Extension with a backhand shot in tennis

Ball and socket joints

Flexion and extension

Flexion and **extension** also occurs in ball and socket joints, including those at the **hip**.

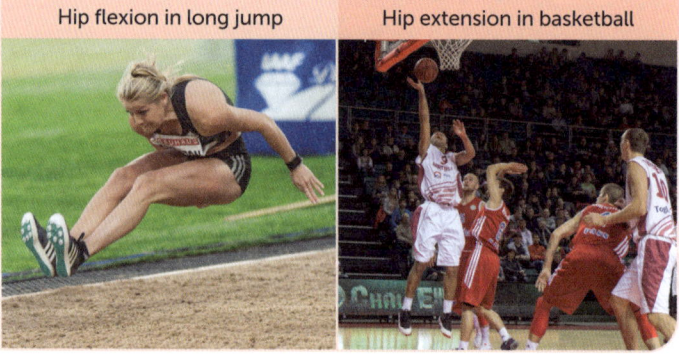

Hip flexion in long jump

Hip extension in basketball

Abduction and adduction

Abduction and **adduction** at the shoulder means to take your arms away (to abduct) from the body, or bringing them back towards (to adduct) the midline of the body. A star jump uses both abduction and adduction.

Abduction in butterfly swimming

Adduction in pull-ups on the rings

⋯ Ball and socket joints continued

Rotation and circumduction

Rotation of the shoulder creates a twisting of the bone along its long axis, such as when you rotate your palm up towards the sky.

Circumduction (think circumference) means a wide circular movement of a limb around the ball and socket joint.

The two movements are often combined.

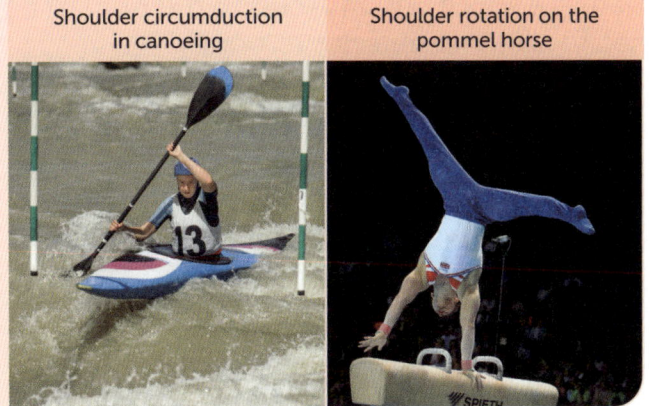

Shoulder circumduction in canoeing

Shoulder rotation on the pommel horse

---

1. Give **three** types of movement which are involved for circumduction around a joint. [3]
2. Analyse the sequence of golfing positions shown in Figure 1.

   Figure 1

   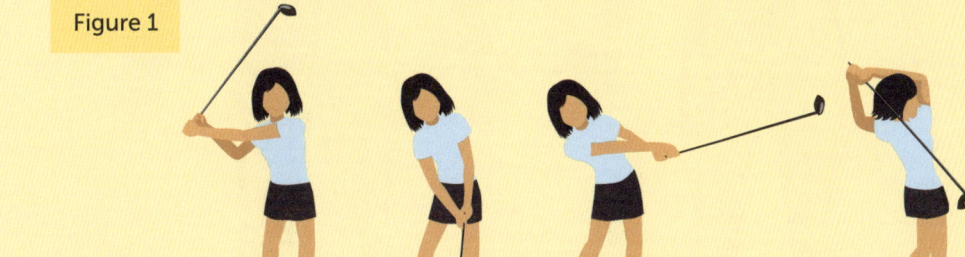

   A   B   C   D

   Describe **two** types of movement taking place at named joints during the golf swing. [4]

---

1. Three from: Flexion,[1] extension,[1] abduction,[1] adduction[1] and rotation.[1]
2. Answers may include:

   Flexion of the arms to start the swing,[1] extending through the swing in positions B and C[1] and flexing again in the follow through in position D.

   Flexion of the hips into the shot in positions A and B[1] with extension in position D[1] of the follow through.

   Abduction of the right arm in position A,[1] adducting through the swing in position B.[1]

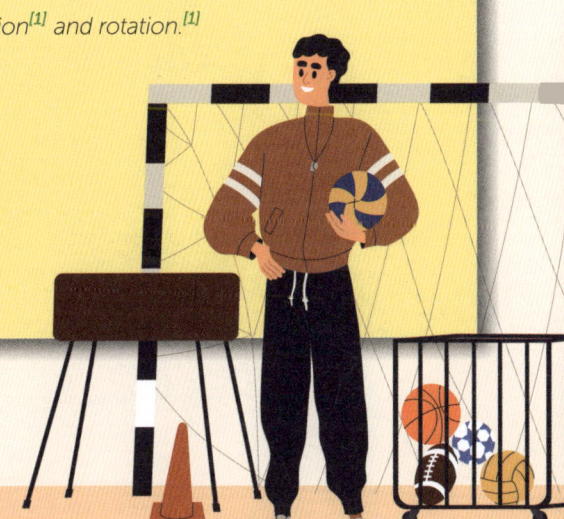

OCR GCSE **Physical Education** – Topic 1.1

1.1.b

LOCATION OF MAJOR MUSCLE GROUPS

There are about 600 **muscles** in the human body. **Tendons** are strong tissue used to connect muscles to bones.

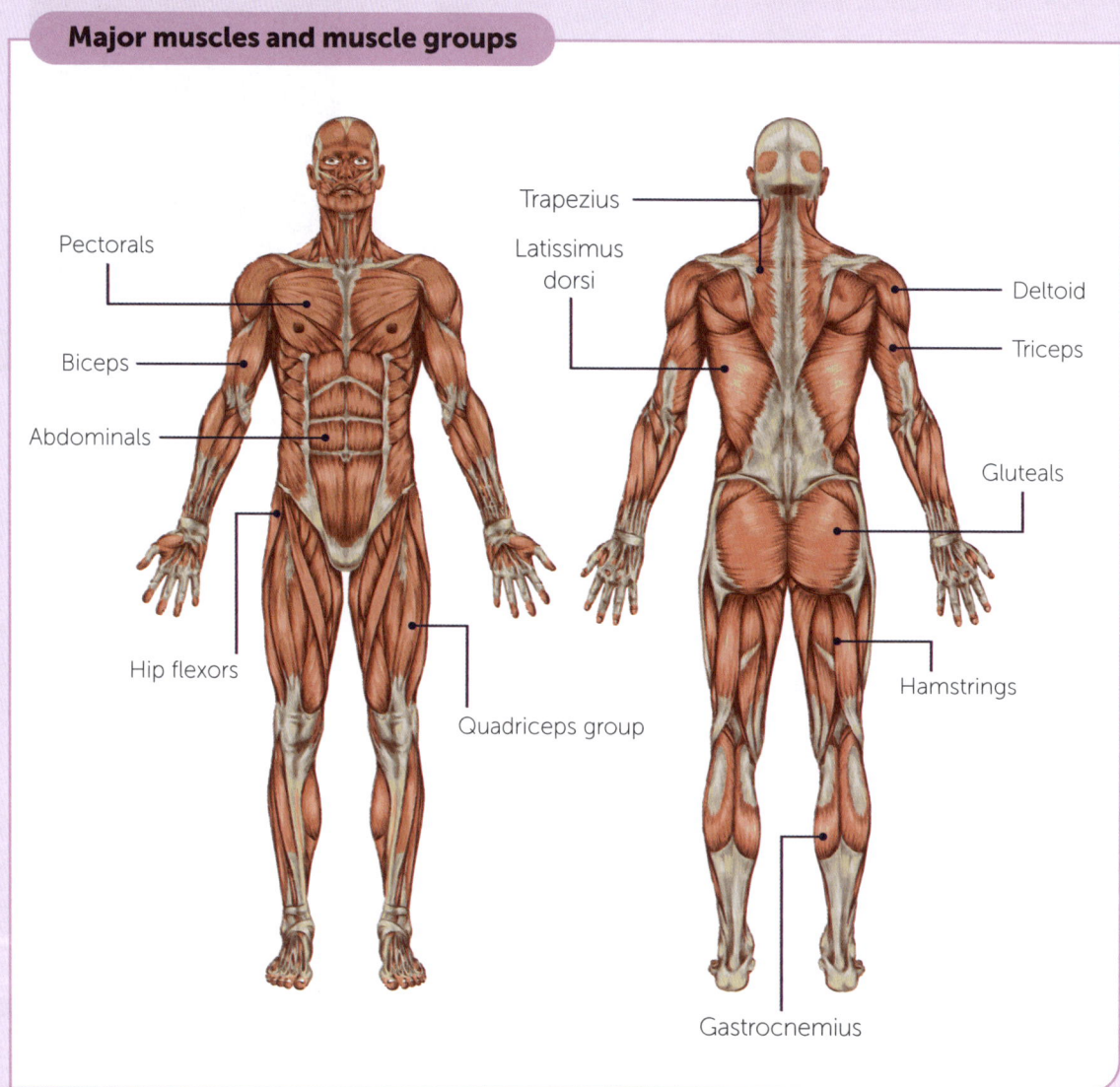

1. Name the leg muscle that contracts during the upward phase of a squat. [1]
2. Name **one** of the primary muscles in the upper body involved in throwing a ball. [1]

1. Quadriceps.[1] (Or one of rectus femoris, vastus medialis, vastus lateralis, vastus intermedius.)
2. Tricep,[1] pectorals,[1] deltoids.[1]

1.1.b

THE ROLES OF MUSCLE IN MOVEMENT

The major muscles of the body work in **antagonistic** pairs. As one muscle (the **agonist**) contracts to pull a bone, the opposite muscle (the **antagonist**) relaxes, to allow the bone to be pulled. This allows movements to take place and sporting actions to be executed.

Antagonistic muscle pairs

The major muscles and muscle groups working together at each major joint are the:

Shoulder:	**Latissimus dorsi** and **deltoid**
Elbow:	**Biceps** and **triceps**
Hip:	**Hip flexors** and **gluteals**
Knee:	**Hamstrings** and **quadriceps**
Ankle:	**Tibialis anterior** and **gastrocnemius**

Agonists are the first muscle to start a movement (the **prime movers**). While the agonist (think pain and agony) contracts, the antagonist relaxes. The bicep is the agonist muscle in the upwards phase of a pull-up, but the antagonist in the upwards phase of a press-up.

Fixator muscles

A **fixator** muscle stabilises the joint, body part or limb to prevent unintended movements. It helps the agonist to work effectively.

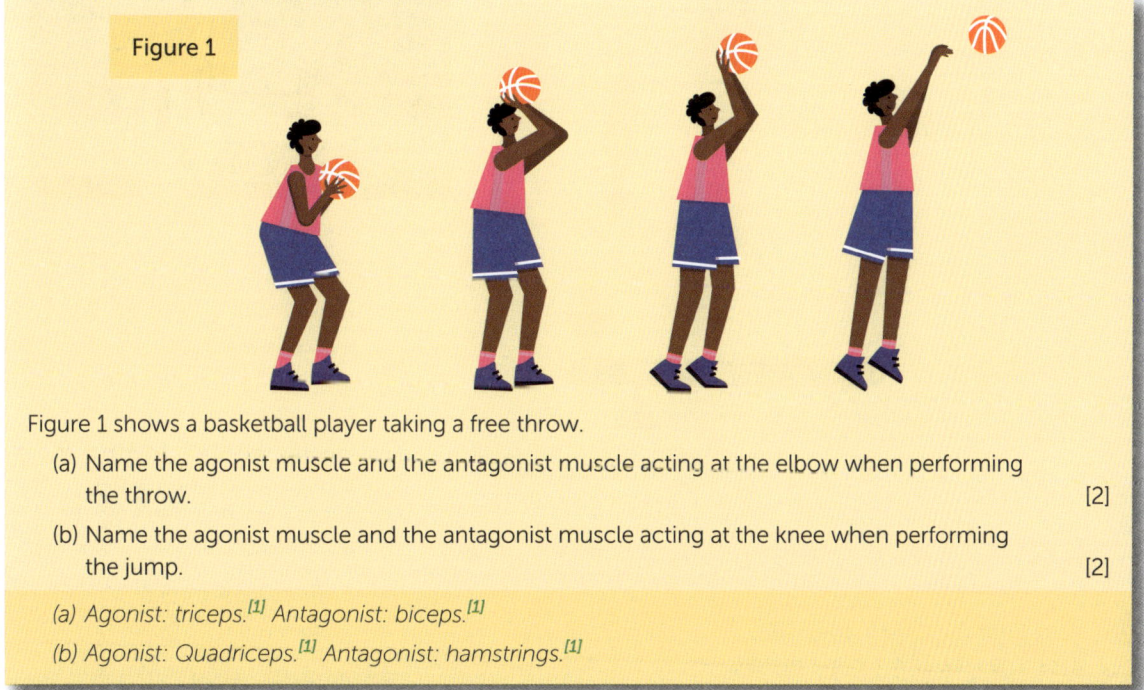

Figure 1

Figure 1 shows a basketball player taking a free throw.
(a) Name the agonist muscle and the antagonist muscle acting at the elbow when performing the throw. [2]
(b) Name the agonist muscle and the antagonist muscle acting at the knee when performing the jump. [2]

(a) Agonist: triceps.[1] Antagonist: biceps.[1]
(b) Agonist: Quadriceps.[1] Antagonist: hamstrings.[1]

1.1.c

LEVER SYSTEMS

There are three classes of lever system in the body. Each lever system has a fulcrum, load and effort.

Fulcrums, load and effort

Levers involve a rigid bar (bone) that pivots or rotates about a fulcrum (joint) with a load applied. A lever system comprises:

- A **fulcrum** or pivot around which a force is exerted. (In the body, this is a joint.)
- A **load** (or **resistance**) being moved. (In the body this relates to bodyweight and any additional load being carried.)
- The **effort** or force required to move the load. (Muscular effort.)

First, second and third class lever systems

First class lever

First class levers have the fulcrum between the effort and the load or resistance, like a see-saw.

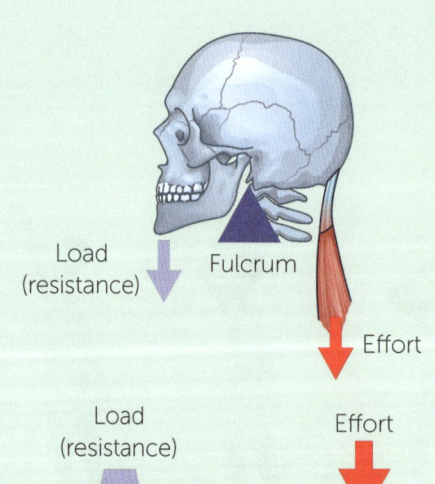

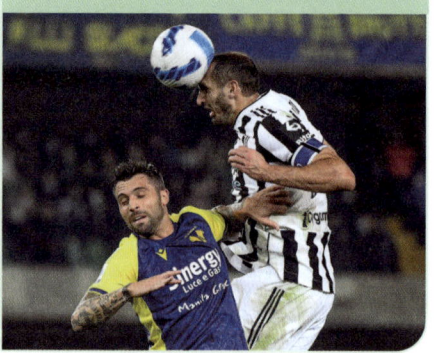

A football player heads a ball using a class 1 lever action in a Serie A Juventus game.

FLE 123 is a useful mnemonic to remember the lever classes.
A class 1 has the *Fulcrum* in the middle.
A class 2 has the *Load* in the middle
A class 3 has the *Effort* in the middle.

1. Complete the statement: The type of lever system working at the knee in the upward phase of a squat is an example of a _____. [1]
2. Identify the lever system that is used to go up onto the toes when pushing off the blocks in a sprint start. [1]

1. Third class lever.[1]
2. Second class lever.[1]

First, second and third class lever systems continued

Second class lever

Second class levers are most easily remembered as having a wheelbarrow action. The fulcrum is at one end with the effort at the opposite end. The load or resistance is anywhere in the middle.

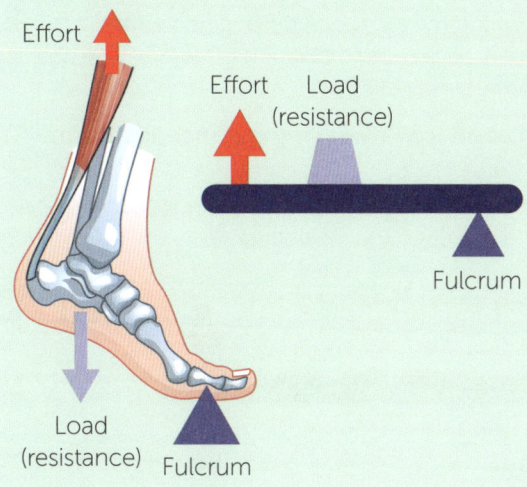

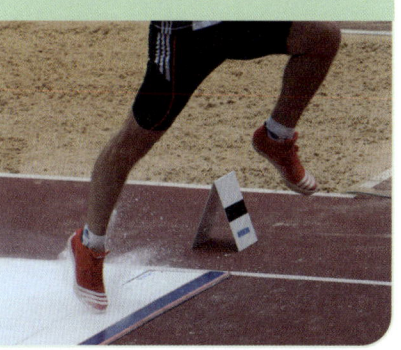

An athlete takes advantage of a class 2 lever action with plantar flexion at the ankle to leave the take off board with explosive power at long jump event.

Think about where the muscle attaches to the bone when considering what type of lever system applies to an action.

Third class lever

A class 3 lever has the fulcrum at one end, the load at the opposite end and the effort applied in the middle.

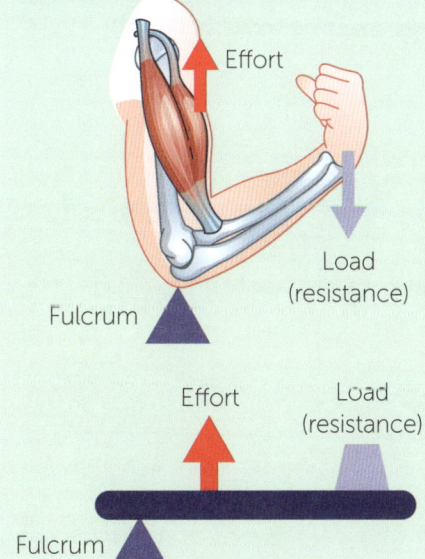

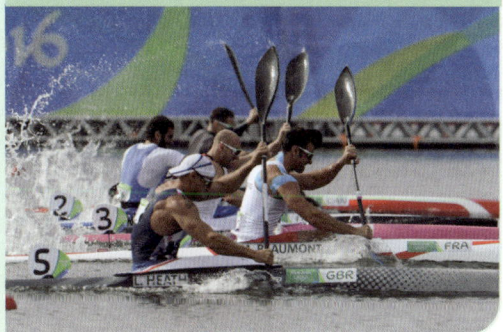

A GB rower uses his biceps to flex at the elbow in a class 3 lever action to draw the paddle through the water in the Men's Kayak Sprint 200m at the Olympic Games in Rio.

OCR GCSE **Physical Education** – Topic 1.1

MECHANICAL ADVANTAGE

A lever is a very simple way to gain mechanical advantage (MA), making lifting or moving much easier.

Calculating mechanical advantage

A lever has a mechanical advantage if its effort arm is longer than its load arm. By comparing the distance of the effort and the load from the fulcrum, you can determine the degree of mechanical advantage. A lever with mechanical advantage is a more efficient lever and will be able to move heavier loads with relatively little effort.

Mechanical advantage = effort arm ÷ weight (resistance/load) arm

A **first class lever** must have the fulcrum nearer to the load than the effort for it to have a mechanical advantage. The nearer it is, the greater the advantage.

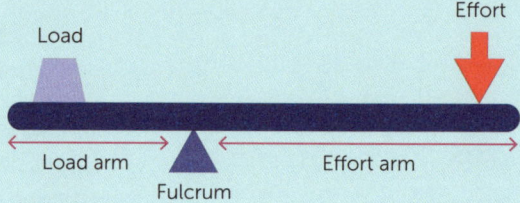

A **second class lever** always has a mechanical advantage of greater than 1 as the effort is always further from the fulcrum than the load. This means a heavy load can be lifted more efficiently.

A **third class lever** is said to have a **mechanical disadvantage** as the effort is always closer to the fulcrum than the load. Despite a mechanical disadvantage when it comes to load, class 3 levers increase distance, so a short muscle movement produces a greater output movement. The hip joint is an example of a class 3 lever, producing large movements of the femur with a relatively small movement near the fulcrum (ball joint).

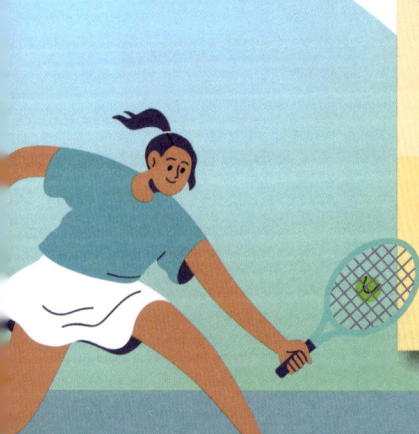

A tennis player makes a backhand volley.
  (a) Identify the type of lever acting in the extension of the elbow during the stroke. [1]
  (b) Explain the mechanical advantage or disadvantage of this lever system. [3]

(a) First class lever.[1]

(b) A mechanical disadvantage occurs[1] as the effort (tricep muscle) is closer to the fulcrum[1] (elbow) than the load[1] (tennis racket in the hand at the end of the forearm). However, a short tricep movement creates a large forearm movement to hit the ball with force.[1]

PLANES OF MOVEMENT AND AXES OF ROTATION

There are three planes and three axes of movement used whilst performing sporting actions.

Planes and axes

A **plane** of movement is an imaginary flat surface across which the body moves in an action. An **axis** of movement is an imaginary line through the body, about which the body rotates.

Movements occur *in* a plane and *around* an axis, so the plane and the axis for a movement should be revised together as pairs.

Sagittal & transverse

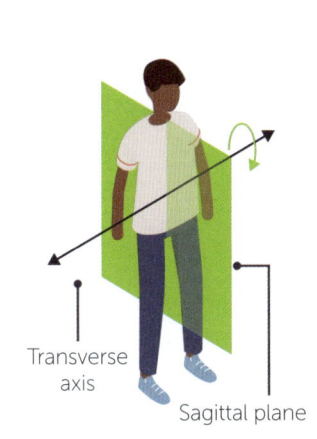

Frontal & frontal

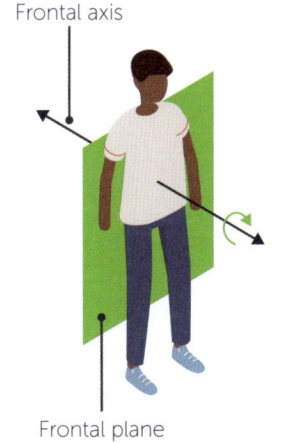

Transverse & Longitudinal

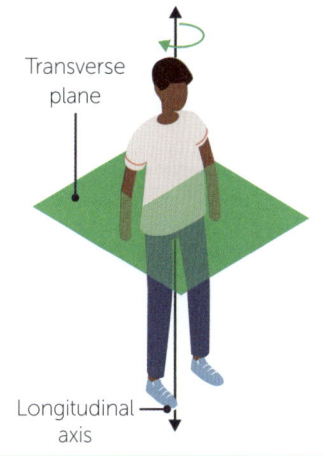

Typical movements

Running, flexion and extension actions take place in the **sagittal plane**.

Bending and rolling actions take place around the **transverse axis**.

Typical movements

Sidestepping and sideways adduction and abduction use the **frontal plane**.

Cartwheels take place around the **frontal axis**.

Typical movements

Twisting, rotating or spinning actions happen in the **transverse plane**.

Spinning and pivoting happen around the **longitudinal axis**.

Figure 1 shows a discus thrower. Identify the plane and axis of movement used in throwing the discus. [2]

Transverse plane. [1]
Longitudinal axis. [1]

Figure 1

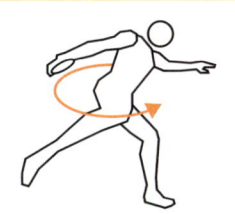

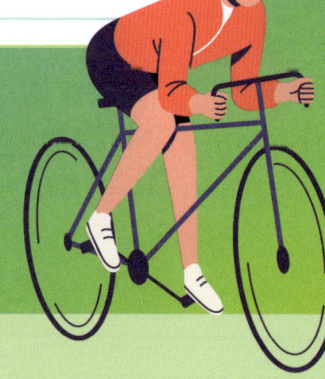

OCR GCSE **Physical Education** – Topic 1.1

STRUCTURE OF THE HEART

The **heart** is an organ that pumps blood around the body using a **double circulatory system**.

The heart

Double circulatory system

A double circulatory system involves two circuits in a complete cycle. The **pulmonary loop** pumps blood between the heart and the lungs for gas exchange to happen, oxygenating the blood and removing CO_2.

The **systemic loop** controls blood flow around the rest of the body to provide organs and working muscles with oxygen and to remove waste products.

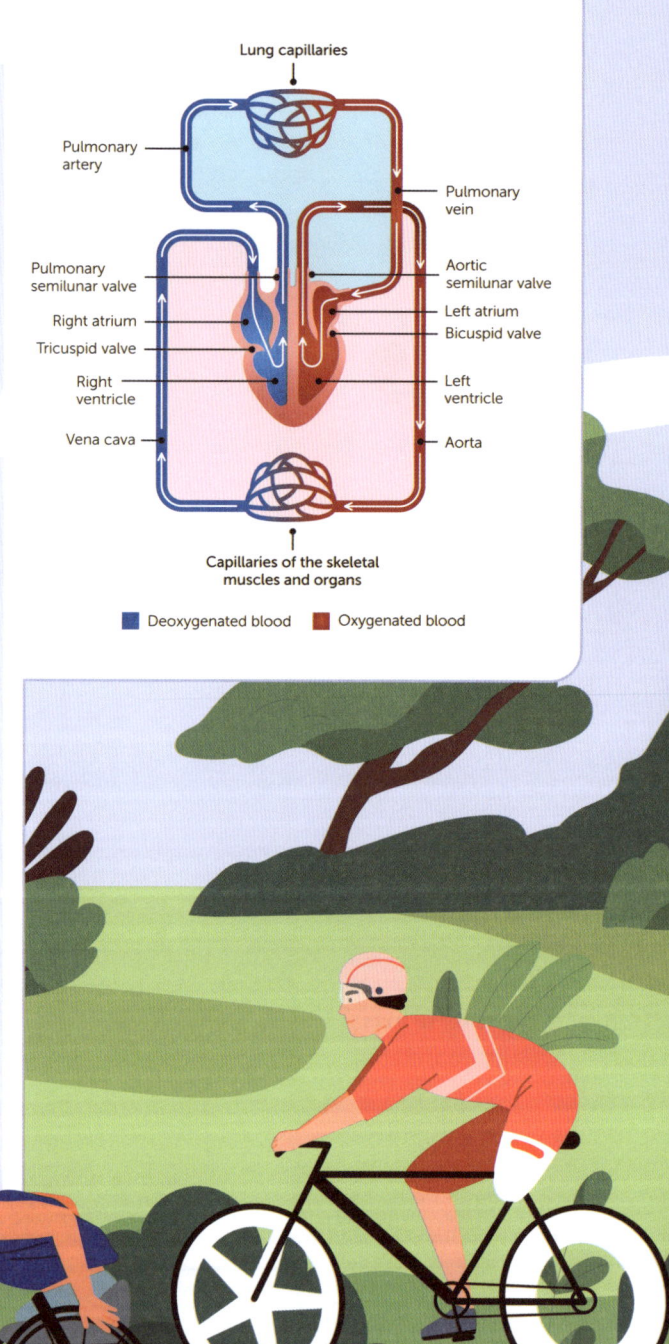

Function of the heart

The heart has walls made of cardiac muscle with **four chambers** and four valves inside. The left and right sections are separated by the **septum** to ensure that oxygenated and deoxygenated blood do not mix.

The **right ventricle** pumps deoxygenated blood around the pulmonary loop to the lungs, where gas exchange takes place. (See page 18.) The **left ventricle** pumps blood around the rest of the body in the systemic loop. The **atria** collect blood as it returns to the heart and pump it into the ventricles. The atria contract together just before the ventricles contract. Oxygen-rich blood is carried away from the heart through **arteries**.

Blood that has given up its oxygen to body cells is carried back to the heart through **veins** – it is deoxygenated. The blood shown as red has been oxygenated in the lungs. **Valves** between the atria and ventricles, and as the blood exits the heart, open and close with pressure, to prevent blood flowing backwards.

1. Complete the figure to show the pathway of the blood around the heart. [5]

   Starting at the vena cava, reorder statements 2–6 to show the pathway of the blood:

   1. Deoxygenated blood fills the right atrium — `1`
   ↓
   2. Then into the left ventricle through the bicuspid valve — [ ]
   ↓
   3. Gas exchange occurs (blood is oxygenated) — [ ]
   ↓
   4. It then flows into the right ventricle — [ ]
   ↓
   5. Pulmonary vein transports oxygenated blood back to the left atrium — [ ]
   ↓
   6. The pulmonary artery then transports deoxygenated blood to the lungs — [ ]
   ↓
   7. Oxygenated blood is ejected and transported to the body via the aorta. — `7`

   1. One mark for each statement in the correct order: 1, 4,[1] 6,[1] 3,[1] 5,[1] 2,[1] 7.

2. Give **two** benefits of a double circulatory system. [2]

   2. Passing through the heart twice allows a higher pressure to be maintained[1] increasing blood flow to the tissues.[1] Ensures oxygenated and deoxygenated blood do not mix.[1]

The role of red blood cells

Red blood cells (or erythrocytes) contain haemoglobin which enables them to carry oxygen. They also carry nutrients around the body. A large surface area increases the speed of diffusion (gas exchange) as they pass through the lungs.

3. Describe **one** role of red blood cells during exercise. [1]

   During exercise, the cells transport oxygen from the lungs to the working muscles of the body.[1] They also transport waste carbon dioxide (CO_2) from the muscles back to the lungs where it can be exhaled.[1]

OCR GCSE **Physical Education** – Topic 1.1

1.1.d

BLOOD VESSELS

The body contains three different types of blood vessel: **arteries**, **veins** and **capillaries**.

The aorta branches into different arteries that carry blood to the major organs. These branch more and more until they form tiny vessels within tissues called capillaries which wrap around muscles and organs. Capillaries then join up to form veins.

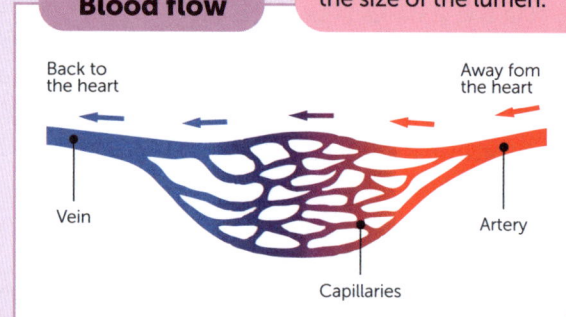

Note that the muscle in arteries does **NOT** pump blood, it simply adjusts the size of the lumen.

Blood vessel structure and function

	Arteries	Capillaries	Veins
Function	Carry **oxygenated** blood at high pressure away from the heart	Exchange of substances with cells	Return **deoxygenated** blood at low pressure to the heart
Lumen	Narrow to maintain pressure	Very narrow. Keeps red blood cells close to tissue cells	Large, so there is less resistance to blood flow
Wall	Elastic fibres stretch and recoil to maintain pressure. Thick wall resists bursting	Very thin – Short distance across to maximise **gas exchange** by diffusion	Low pressure so no need for a thick elastic wall
Valve	No – High pressure blood keeps moving	No	Yes – Prevents backflow of low pressure blood

1. Define what is meant by a blood vessel. [1]
2. "All arteries carry oxygenated blood. All veins carry deoxygenated blood."
   Is this statement true or false? [1]

---

1. A tubular structure that carries blood around the body.[1]
2. False.[1] All arteries carry blood from the heart and veins carry it toward the heart but the pulmonary vein carries oxygenated blood to the heart from the lungs and the pulmonary artery carries deoxygenated blood to the lungs to be oxygenated.

HEART RATE, STROKE VOLUME AND CARDIAC OUTPUT

Heart rate and stroke volume

Heart rate is the frequency with which the heart contracts (beats). It is measured in **beats per minute**. The natural resting heart rate is controlled by a group of cells found in the right atrium. They act as a pacemaker, producing regular impulses that travel through the heart causing it to contract.

Heart rate naturally increases during exercise to supply the muscles with the additional oxygen they need. Before exercise, adrenaline will cause the heart rate to rise in anticipation.

Stroke volume is the volume of blood pumped out of the heart by the left ventricle with one contraction.

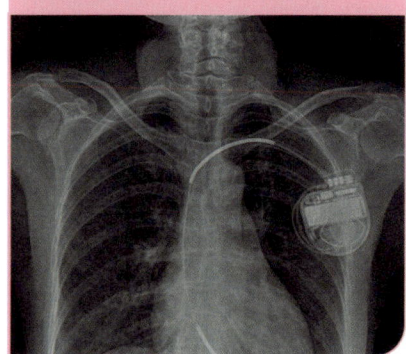

Artificial pacemakers are electrical devices used to correct irregularities in the heart rate.

Cardiac output

The volume of blood pumped by each ventricle of the heart in one minute is called the cardiac output. It is calculated as the product of stroke volume and the heart rate.

Cardiac output (Q) = stroke volume (mL) × heart rate (beats per minute)

1. A person has a resting stroke volume of 60 ml/beat and a heart rate of 65 beats per minute (bpm). Calculate the cardiac output. [2]
2. The following heart rate graph shows the data from a cyclist's training session.
    (a) Explain why the heart rate increased before exercise began at 8 mins. [2]
    (b) Suggest what might have caused a changed in heart rate at 13 mins and 17 mins. [1]

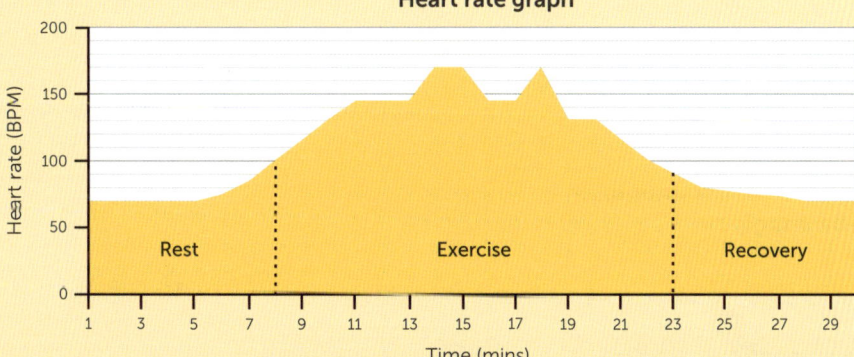

1. 60 × 65 = 3900[1] mL per minute / 3.9 litres per minute.[1]
2. (a) Before exercise, adrenaline[1] will cause an anticipatory[1] rise in heart rate.
    (b) A hill / greater resistance[1] could create a more intense period of exertion.

OCR GCSE **Physical Education** – Topic 1.1

STRUCTURE AND FUNCTION OF THE RESPIRATORY SYSTEM

The pathway of air

1. As you breathe, air is drawn in through the **nose or mouth** into the **trachea**.
2. It passes into the **bronchi**,
3. ...and branches into the smaller **bronchioles**,
4. ...which fills the **lungs**,
5. ...where oxygen is diffused into the blood via smaller air sacs called **alveoli**.

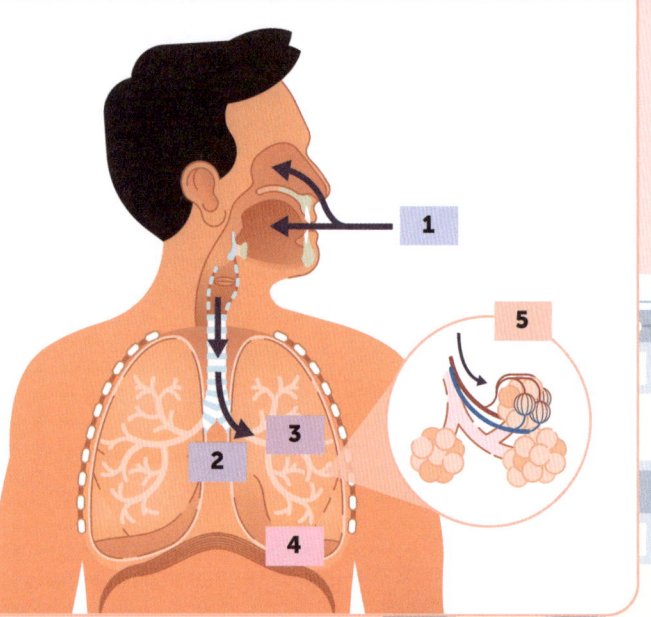

Gaseous exchange

The **alveoli** provide a very large surface area with **moist**, **thin** walls only **one cell thick**. This makes **diffusion** easier as the distance across one cell is so short. Lots of blood **capillaries** create a **strong blood supply** for the oxygen to diffuse into.

Two gases diffusing in opposite directions at the same time is called **gaseous exchange**. **Oxygen concentration** is lower in the capillaries than it is in the alveoli, so it passes through the capillary membrane into the blood until an equilibrium is reached through diffusion. **Carbon dioxide** in the capillaries is in greater concentration than in the alveoli so it passes back through the other way into the lungs to be exhaled.

Oxygen combines with **haemoglobin** in the red blood cells to form **oxyhaemoglobin**. Haemoglobin can also carry carbon dioxide.

Gaseous exchange also takes place in the muscles where oxygen passes from the bloodstream to the muscles.

1. Explain how oxygen and carbon dioxide swap between the lungs and the bloodstream. [2]

    1. The concentration of each gas will try equalise on both sides of the alveolo–capillary membrane.[1] so where there is greater concentration of one gas on one side, some will pass through to provide more oxygen in the blood or to remove excess carbon dioxide.[1]

The role of respiratory muscles in breathing

Changes in air pressure cause inhalation and exhalation. The rate of inhalation and exhalation can be controlled through the use of chest and abdominal muscles such as the **rib cage**, **intercostal muscles** (those between the ribs) and the **diaphragm**.

When inhaling, negative air pressure is created within the lungs to draw in a breath of air. Air always moves from areas of high pressure to areas of low pressure to create an equilibrium of pressure.

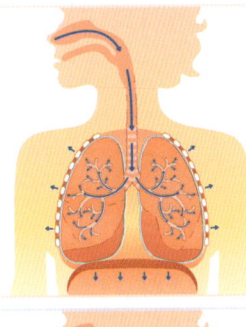

Inhalation
1. The diaphragm contracts, moving downwards from a dome shape to a flatter shape.
2. The intercostal muscles contract moving the rib cage up and out.
3. This increases the volume inside the chest cavity;
4. Which decreases the pressure inside the chest cavity.
5. A pressure gradient is created, pulling air into the lungs through the nose or mouth.

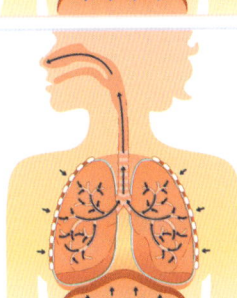

Exhalation
1. The diaphragm relaxes and returns to a dome shape.
2. The intercostal muscles relax moving the rib cage down and back.
3. This decreases the volume inside the chest cavity;
4. Which increases the pressure inside the chest cavity.
5. A pressure gradient is created and air is pushed out.

The effect of exercise on breathing

During exercise, inhalation and exhalation needs to happen more quickly to allow the lungs to diffuse more oxygen into the bloodstream. The lungs can also expand more on **inspiration** (breathing in) with the use of the **pectoral muscles** and **sternocleidomastoid**.

During **expiration** (breathing out), the rib cage is pulled down to force air out more quickly with use of the **abdominal muscles**.

2. Complete the table by adding **one** tick to each row to show how each of the following skeletal muscles help in the breathing process during exercise. [3]

Muscle	Helps with inhalation?	Helps with exhalation?
Abdominals		
Pectoral muscles		
Sternocleidomastoid		

2. Inhalation: pectoral[1] muscles and sternocleidomastoid.[1] Exhalation: abdominals.[1]

BREATHING RATE AND TIDAL VOLUME

A **spirometer** is a device used to measure lung volumes, such as the amount of air inhaled and exhaled in each breath. A device reading is called a **trace**.

Lung volume measurements at rest and during exercise

Tidal volume

Tidal volume is the volume of air inhaled or exhaled per breath. At rest, tidal volume is approximately 500ml.

Respiratory rate

Respiratory rate is the number of breaths taken in one minute.

Minute ventilation

Minute ventilation is the volume of air that is inhaled or exhaled in 60 seconds. It is calculated from the product of the **tidal volume** and the **respiratory rate**.

Minute ventilation = tidal volume (mL) × respiratory rate

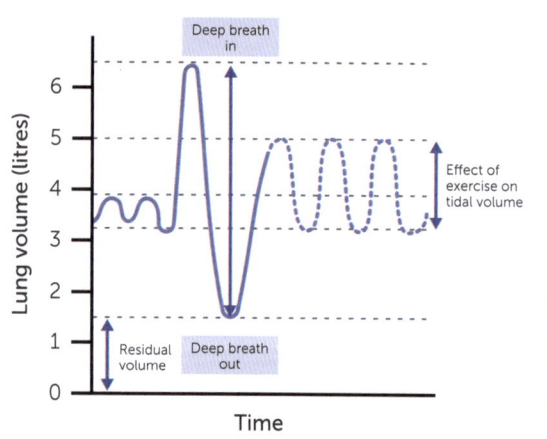

A spirometer trace.

Exercise can change the volume of air required by a performer.

(a) Describe the effect of exercise on the tidal volume. [1]

(b) Explain how long-term exercise and fitness training may impact minute ventilation. [1]

(a) The tidal volume will increase,[1] as more oxygen is required by the working muscles.

(b) Maximum minute ventilation will increase during exercise as lung capacity increases.[1] Resting minute ventilation may remain the same or reduce slightly[1] as the body produces more alveoli and becomes more efficient at extracting oxygen from the air.

1.1.d

AEROBIC AND ANAEROBIC EXERCISE

Aerobic exercise means being in the presence of, or using oxygen.
Anaerobic exercise occurs when the heart and lungs cannot supply blood and oxygen to muscles as fast as the respiring cells need them.

Aerobic exercise

Aerobic capacity is the ability to take in and transfer oxygen to the working muscles in order to exercise continuously without tiring. During **aerobic exercise**, like marathon running, the relatively **low intensity** of the activity should allow for the heart and lungs to provide enough oxygen for the muscles to use as they work. As a result, the activity can be sustained for a **long period** of time (duration). Examples include:

- Marathon running
- 2000m rowing
- Distance cycling
- Gentle skipping

Oxygen mixes with the glucose in the body to produce energy to fuel muscle movement. Waste products are water (sweat) and carbon dioxide (through increased exhalation).

Summary of aerobic exercise:

(glucose + oxygen → energy + carbon dioxide + water)

Anaerobic exercise

During **anaerobic** exercise, like sprinting, the **high intensity** of the activity doesn't allow the heart and lungs to provide enough oxygen for the muscles to use as they work. The activity is too intense for delivery to keep up with demand. As a result, muscles are forced to work without enough oxygen and **lactic acid** is produced as a waste product. The lactic acid causes pain and fatigue so these activities can only be sustained for a **short period** of time (duration). Examples include:

- Sprinting
- Heavy weightlifting
- Cycling sprints
- Long jump

Summary of anaerobic exercise:

(glucose → energy + lactic acid)

The **duration** and/or **intensity** of a physical activity generally determine if it is aerobic or anaerobic. Anaerobic activity is usually for less than a minute.

Discuss whether swimming should be considered aerobic or anaerobic. [6]

A 10k swim would be performed over a long period of time[✓] with moderate exertion throughout and little or no opportunity to rest[✓] which is aerobic.[✓] Sufficient oxygen would be available for energy to be produced to maintain muscle contractions.[✓]

A competitive 50m race would be of high intensity and could not be sustained for long.[✓] Lactic acid would be produced by the muscles owing to a lack of oxygen[✓] which is anaerobic[✓] as the blood uses its own blood sugar and/or glycogen stores as an alternative energy source given the lack of oxygen.[✓] Depending on the intensity of the swimming, and the period of time over which it is done, it could be either.[✓] *This question should be marked in accordance with the levels of response guidance on page 99.*

1.1.e

THE SHORT-TERM EFFECTS OF EXERCISE

The effects of exercise on muscles and bones, the heart and the respiratory system depend on the period over which activity is undertaken.

Short-term effects of exercise on the body

Muscle temperature

Muscles generate heat as they create energy. Exercise also increases blood flow to the working muscles increasing their temperature. Warming muscles makes them more **elastic** so that they are more likely to **stretch** rather than tear.

Heart rate, stroke volume and cardiac output

During exercise, the heart rate, stroke volume and cardiac output will increase to pump newly oxygenated blood to the working muscles and to remove waste carbon dioxide.

Redistribution of blood flow during exercise (Vascular shunting)

When exercising, the body redistributes blood to increase flow to the muscles that most need the oxygen it carries. This is known as the **vascular shunt** mechanism. The body increases the width of the arteries, known as **vasodilation**, to increase flow to skeletal muscles. **Vasoconstriction** is the term given to the narrowing of blood vessels to restrict blood flow to tissues and organs (such as the liver, gut and kidneys) that are not vital during maximal exercise. Blood is shunted back to the organs when exercise pauses or stops.

1. The table below shows the redistribution of blood during exercise.

Destination	Rest	Maximal exercise
Skeletal muscles	19%	86%
Major internal organs	71%	8%
Skin	10%	6%

(a) Using the data in the table, analyse the redistribution of blood to the skin during exercise. [1]
(b) Give **one** reason why the distribution of blood is necessary. [1]
(c) Explain why the skin becomes hot and red during intense exercise. [2]

(a) It decreases[1] (by 4%).
(b) To supply the skeletal muscles with the increased oxygen / nutrients they need during exercise.[1] To regulate body temperature.[1]
(c) Hot, sweaty, red skin is caused by an increase in temperature as a result of lost energy,[1] and the dilation of blood vessels below the skin to reduce body temperature.[1] Whilst there is a decrease in the percentage of blood flow distributed to the skin during exercise, the amount of blood flow increases.[1]

Short-term effects on the body continued

Respiratory rate, tidal volume and minute ventilation

Exercise causes the respiratory rate, tidal volume and minute ventilation to increase. The increase in the depth and frequency of breathing happens to bring more air (and therefore oxygen) into the lungs to oxygenate the blood more quickly. Increased exhalation also removes waste carbon dioxide more quickly.

Supplying oxygen to the working muscles

The working muscles demand more oxygen-rich blood during exercise. In response to this demand, the heart works harder to pump blood to the working muscles more quickly, and blood pressure increases. Vascular shunting (see left) also redirects blood to the muscles during exercise and reduces the flow to the major organs to a minimal level.

Lactic acid production

Working muscles produce **blood lactate** (lactic acid) and carbon dioxide as waste products during vigorous exercise. Increased blood flow improves the supply of oxygen to the muscles to reduce the build up of lactic acid and also helps to carry away lactic acid and CO_2 that has already accumulated. Lactic acid causes fatigue in the muscles which is experienced as pain and discomfort, reducing performance and causing heart rate to stay higher than normal.

2. Figure 2 below shows the respiratory rate of a rugby player before, during and after a match.

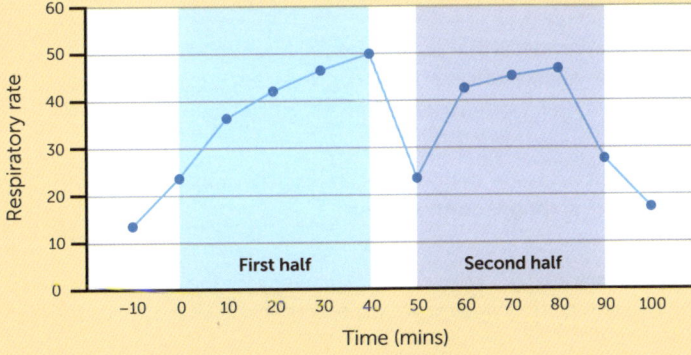

Figure 2

(a) Using the information in the graph, analyse how the respiratory rates compare in the first half and second half of the game and give reasons for their difference. [3]

(b) Explain why the respiratory rate dropped significantly between 40 and 50 minutes. [1]

(a) First half became more intense than the second half.[1] First half got gradually more intense as the match progressed but the second half was consistently intense until the last 10 minutes.[1] Performance in the first half was intense until the whistle but the second half tailed off 10 minutes before the end.[1] This may be caused by a change in team possession of the ball / change of strategy / decline in motivation / tiredness / injury / time in the sin bin.[1]

(b) Half time break so the player had a lower demand for oxygen.[1]

OCR GCSE **Physical Education** – Topic 1.1

1.1.e

THE LONG-TERM EFFECTS OF EXERCISE

The long-term effects of exercise can make gradual, but significant improvements in specific **components of fitness** (see **pages 29** to **36**). The exact benefits of exercise depend on the type of activities that are undertaken.

Long-term effects of exercise

Increased bone density happens as muscles pull on them creating more work for them, building their strength and thickness. This increases the protection on a performer's skeletal system and internal organs in contact sports. It also helps to reduce **osteoporosis**.

Hypertrophy of muscle means an increase in the size of skeletal muscles, often happening as a result of training or exercise. This could provide a competitive advantage over a smaller performer.

Greater muscular strength can increase power and explosive strength in a rugby game for example.

Increased muscular endurance helps you perform stronger and for longer. The ability to move your body and muscles repeatedly without fatiguing increases with regular exercise. This is especially helpful for endurance athletes and games players.

Greater resistance to fatigue develops as muscles become less tired through greater efficiency of the body to produce energy.

Hypertrophy of the heart results in a stronger, healthier heart reducing the resting heart rate and the risk of heart attacks, angina and coronary heart disease.

Lower resting heart rate (bradycardia) occurs as a healthier, more muscular, heart can achieve a **higher stroke volume**, delivering sufficient oxygen to a resting body with fewer beats and therefore with greater efficiency.

> **Hypertrophy** is the name given to the enlargement of skeletal or cardiac muscle through micro-tears that heal, increasing mass.

Increased cardiac output occurs as a stronger heart results in a thicker wall of the left ventricle which can pump out more blood with **stronger contractions**.

Improved rate of recovery enables a performer to be ready for the next match, event or training more quickly. Lactic acid can also be removed more efficiently through increased cardiac output.

Increased aerobic capacity develops as stronger lungs and heart muscles are able to deliver oxygen to the working muscles more efficiently so a performer can work harder and for longer without tiring.

Stronger respiratory muscles through hypertrophy. The surface area of the alveoli also increases, making gas exchange more efficient.

Increased tidal volume and minute volume happens with regular exercise over months and years of exercise.

Capillarisation is an increase in the number of capillaries as a result of regular exercise over time. The density of capillaries around the alveoli and surrounding muscles increases to facilitate more efficient gas exchange.

1. Explain why cardiac hypertrophy can result in a lower resting heart rate. [2]
2. Paul plays hockey and has tested his fitness in each month of training over a one year period. His results are shown in the graph below.

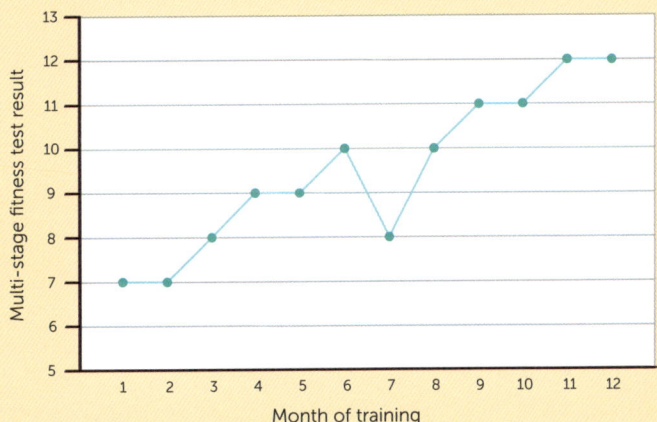

(a) Discuss how the long term effects of exercise on cardiovascular endurance and stamina could be beneficial to Paul. [3]

(b) Give **one** reason why month 7 may have been lower than expected. [1]

1. Cardiac hypertrophy is an increase in the size of the heart[1] which means that stroke volume can increase / more blood is ejected per beat.[1] Increasing the size of the heart[1] means that it can pump an increased volume of blood around the body with each cycle.[1] As the body size remains the same, the heart no longer needs to work as hard to deliver sufficient blood to the organs at rest[1] so the heart rate lowers.[1]

2. (a) Increase in endurance means that Paul is able to perform for a whole match without tiring.[1] Increased rate of removal of lactic acid means that Paul can play harder for longer.[1] A greater resistance to fatigue so Paul can play for longer or player harder.[1] Stronger respiratory muscles help Paul to deliver more oxygen to the working muscles.[1] Hypertrophy of the heart means that Paul may be able to play hockey for more years and reduce his risk of related diseases.[1]

   (b) Reversibility,[1] off day,[1] illness,[1] injury,[1] test taken too soon after match, so insufficient recovery time.[1]

OCR GCSE **Physical Education** – Topic 1.1

Topic 1.1

EXAMINATION PRACTICE

1. Which **one** of the following bones is located at the hip? [1]
   - ☐ A – Femur
   - ☐ B – Scapula
   - ☐ C – Talus
   - ☐ D – Tibia

2. A wide circular movement of the arm around the shoulder joint is an example of circumduction. Is this statement true or false? [1]
   - ☐ True
   - ☐ False

3. Blood flows around the body in a double circulatory system.
   (a) Which **one** of the following describes the correct pathway of the blood as it enters the heart via the pulmonary vein? [1]
   - ☐ A – Left atrium → left ventricle → right atrium → right ventricle
   - ☐ B – Left atrium → right atrium → left ventricle → right atrium
   - ☐ C – Right atrium → right ventricle → left atrium → left ventricle
   - ☐ D – Right ventricle → left ventricle → right atrium → left atrium

   (b) Describe the differences between the aorta and the vena cava. [4]

4. Give **three** functions of the skeleton. [3]

5. Tendons, ligaments and cartilage are found at major synovial joints.
   (a) Explain **two** differences between tendons and ligaments. [2]
   (b) State the function of cartilage in the prevention of pain and injury. [1]

6. Lee conducts a press up into a high plank position.

   Position A   Position B

   (a) Identify the working muscle in the arm above the elbow responsible for the movement from position A to position B. [1]
   (b) Describe the role of the latissimus dorsi as a fixator muscle in a press up. [2]

7. An athlete is shown below, performing a bicep curl.

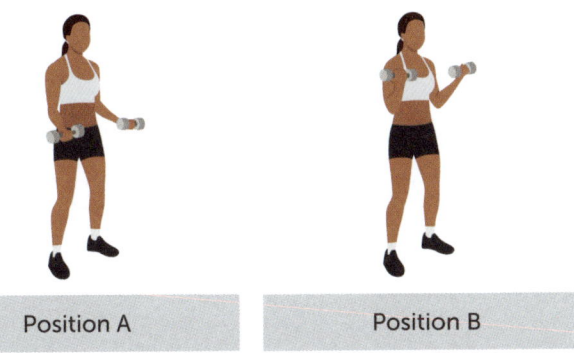

Position A   Position B

(a) Identify the class of lever acting at the elbow during a bicep curl. [1]
(b) Draw a fully labelled diagram to show the class of lever identified in part (a). [2]

8. **Figure A** shows an ice skater rotating on the ice.

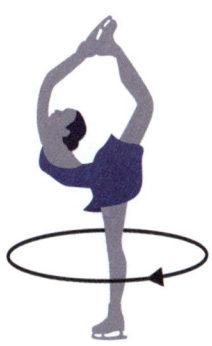

Figure A

(a) (i) Identify the plane and axis of movement used to allow flexion at the knee of the raised leg. [2]
    (ii) Identify the plane and axis of movement used in performing the spin on the ice. [2]

The skater jumps into a spin using a third-class lever at the hip and knee.

(b) Identify the joint movement at the hip and knee of the driving leg on take off in a jump. [1]
(c) Explain why a class three lever has no mechanical advantage. [2]

To maintain balance in Figure A, the skater uses abduction.

(d) Define abduction using an example from Figure A. [1]

9. The effects of exercise depend on the period over which activity is taken.
   (a) Which **one** of the following is short term effect of exercise? [1]

   ☐ A – Improved muscular endurance
   ☐ B – Improved speed
   ☐ C – Increased heart rate
   ☐ D – Increased size of the heart

   (b) Discuss how long-term fitness training can improve an ice skater's performance. [6]

10. Describe how muscles and bones work together to produce movement. [3]

11. Petra plays basketball.

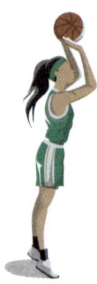

Petra's tidal volume was monitored for one minute before and after the game starts. A graph is shown below.

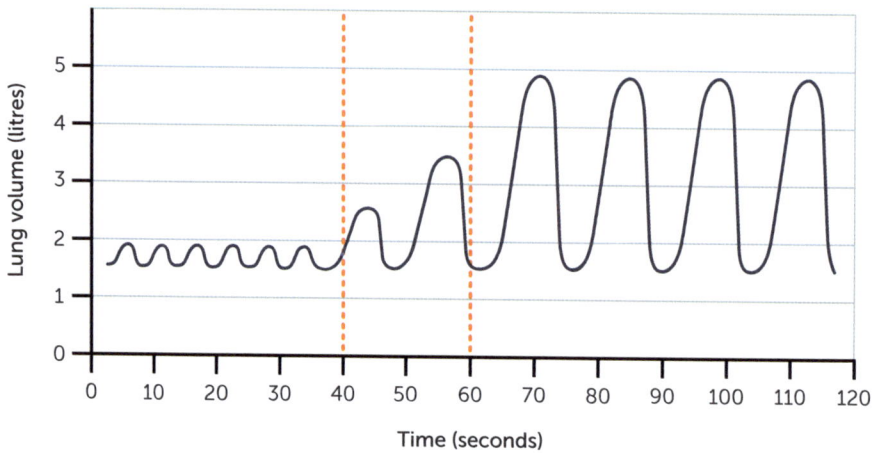

(a) Define what is meant by tidal volume. [1]
(b) At 60 seconds, Petra walks onto the court to play.
Explain the effect of exercise on her tidal volume. [1]
(c) Explain why Petra's tidal volume may have started to change after 40 seconds. [1]
(d) Name **one** muscle that helps Petra diaphragm to take a deeper breath when she needs it during intense exercise. [1]

When Petra takes a breath, air is drawn into her lungs to the alveoli.
(e) Explain the role of Petra's respiratory muscles during inhalation. [4]
(f) Describe the function of the alveoli. [3]
(g) Give **one** advantage to Petra of increasing her cardiovascular endurance or stamina. [1]

THE COMPONENTS OF FITNESS

Each of the components of fitness can be linked to various sports and can help to plan, carry out, monitor and evaluate exercise and training programmes to suit individual needs.

Cardiovascular endurance (stamina)

Cardiovascular endurance or **stamina** is the ability to continue exertion while getting energy from the aerobic system used to supply the body with energy. It can be measured using the Cooper 12 minute run/walk test or the multi-stage fitness test.

Marathon and endurance runners need stamina to be able to maintain a high volume of oxygenated blood to the working muscles for a prolonged period.

Cooper 12 minute run/walk test

Participants of the Cooper test aim to cover as much distance as they can in 12 minutes using a **track**, some **distance markers**, **recording sheets** and a **stopwatch**. Distance is usually measured in kilometres or miles. The test can be carried out on multiple people at the same time.

Expected performance is based on gender and age, but range between a score of 'Excellent' for a distance of over 2800 metres for a male in his twenties, and a score of 'Poor' for 1100 metres by a woman in her fifties.

> Kenneth Cooper MD created the Cooper test in 1968 to measure of the maximum amount of oxygen that a person can use during exercise.
>
> The test is still used in the military for stamina.

Multi-stage fitness test

Cones, an assistant and a measuring tape of at least 20m in length are required to set up the test. An audio player and recording of the bleeps is also required at the start.

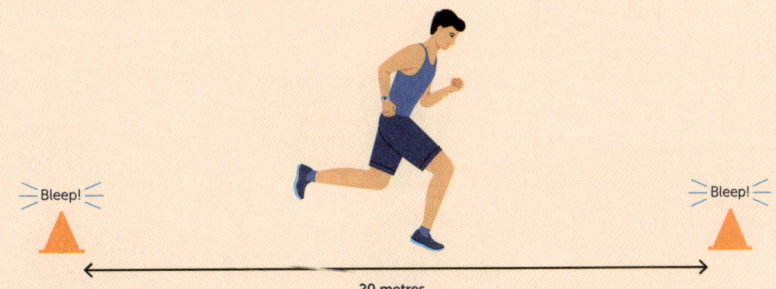

When the assistant begins playing the recording of the bleeps, the participant must run 20 metres to reach the other cone before the next bleep. The time interval between bleeps gets progressively shorter, requiring faster and faster shuttle runs between the cones. Failure to reach the cone before the bleep twice in a row ends the test, and the last properly completed level should be recorded. The score is usually recorded as a level and bleep number, for example 5/7.

Muscular endurance

Muscular endurance is the ability of a muscle or muscle group to undergo repeated contractions, without fatigue. It can be measured using the press-up test or the sit-up test.

Triathletes require muscular endurance for **running**, **swimming** and **cycling** to reduce fatigue in muscles repeatedly contracting. **Canoeists** and **football players** also benefit.

Press-up test

The **press-up test** requires a **flat area** and a **stopwatch**. Using the correct technique, participants start with their arms extended and perform as many press-ups in a minute as they can. Resting is permitted only in the raised position. Performance is measured according to age and gender.

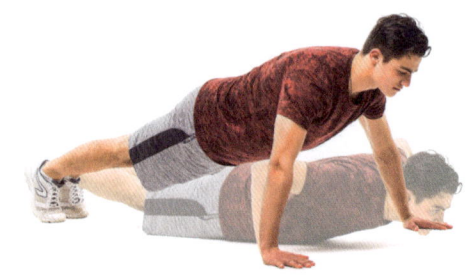

Sit-up test

The **sit-up test** requires a partner to support the feet and ankles, and to press play on an audio recording of progressively faster bleeps. The participant sits up and back down again to the rhythm of the bleeps. As a **maximal test**, the sit ups continue until the participant can no longer keep time with the bleeps. The score is equal to the number of sit ups performed.

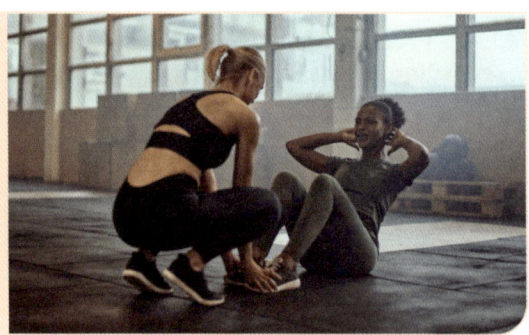

1. Evaluate the use of the press up test for a sprint cyclist. [2]

    1. The test measures the muscular endurance of the upper body and arms only.[1] Sprint cyclists need muscular endurance[1] but they rely on their leg muscles which are not tested using this method.[1]

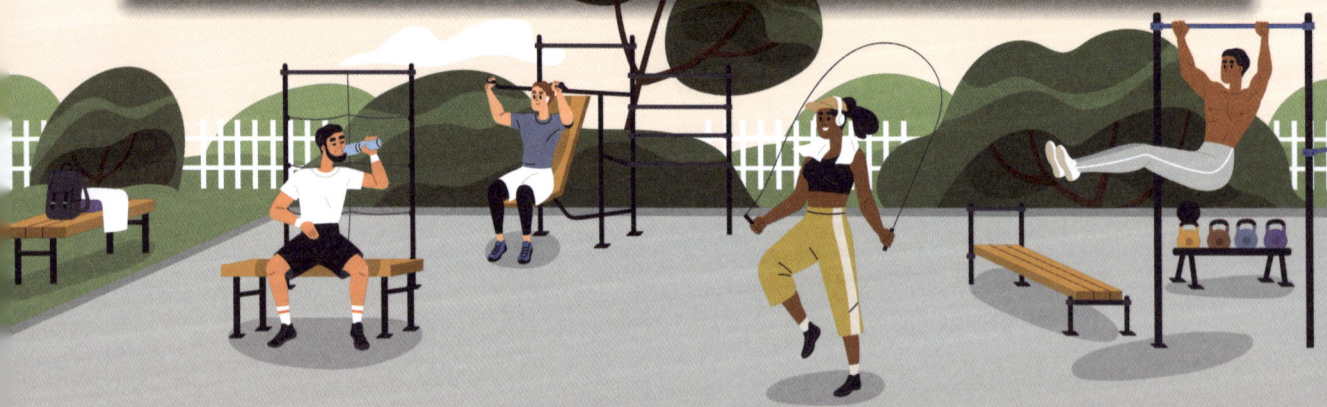

Speed

Speed is the ability to move quickly across the ground or move limbs rapidly through actions. It can be measured using the 30m sprint test.

Sprinters and **tennis players** require speed to move quickly across a track or court.

30m sprint test

2. The 30 metre sprint test measures speed. Describe how to carry out this test. [3]

   2. Use 2 cones and place them 30 metres apart[1] using a tape measure.[1] Allow a flying start to the sprint[1] and with a stop watch, time the athlete running as they pass between the start and end cones.[1] Record the time in seconds.[1]

 Agility

Agility, or nimbleness, is the ability to change direction at speed.

Rugby players need agility to sidestep around the opposition to avoid a tackle and gain territory.

Illinois agility test

This test measures agility.

It requires **eight cones**, carefully arranged at measured distances apart as shown in the diagram. The performer starts face down and runs against a **stopwatch timer** to the end. The activity is measured in seconds.

See **page 48** for national standards.

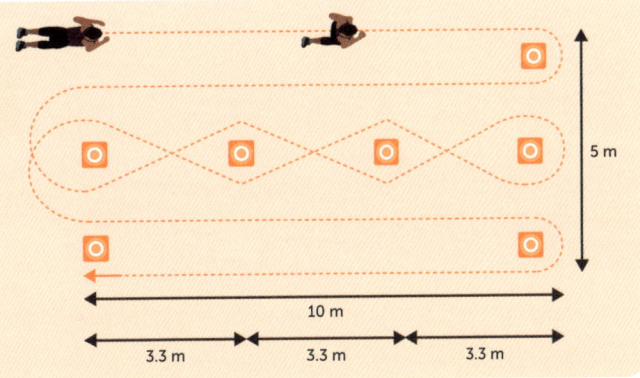

3. Speed and agility are useful in sports that require sudden changes of direction, such as football, hockey and badminton.

Performer	30 metre sprint test (seconds)	Illinois agility test (seconds)
Joe	4.2	15.8
Karl	4.6	16.4
Mason	4.3	16.3

The table above shows some test results for a group of male <18 football players.
(a) Which player appears to be slowest? [1]   (b) Which player has the greatest agility? [1]

3. (a) Karl.[1]   (b) Joe.[1]

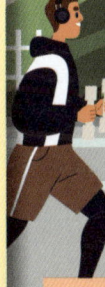

OCR GCSE **Physical Education** – Topic 1.2

Strength

Strength is THE maximum force a muscle, or group of muscles can apply against a resistance. It can be further categorised as maximal, static, dynamic and explosive strength. Strength can be measured using the grip strength dynamometer test or the 1 Repetition Maximum (RM) test.

High maximal strength is required in **boxing** and **weightlifting**. Static strength helps **rugby players** to hold the resistance in a scrum position. **Gymnasts** have high dynamic strength.

Grip strength dynamometer test

This measures **grip strength**. Using a handgrip dynamometer in the dominant hand, squeeze the handle with maximum effort keeping the elbow at 90 degrees. Record the best score.

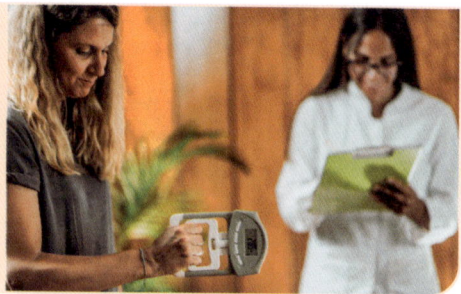

1 Repetition Maximum (1RM) test

The **1 rep max test** measures the maximal weight that can be lifted in a single attempt. Using free weights or a specialised machine and a spotter, a participant should select a suitable weight and lift it once using the correct technique. After a few minutes rest, they should increase the weight and try again, repeating this until they reach their maximum.

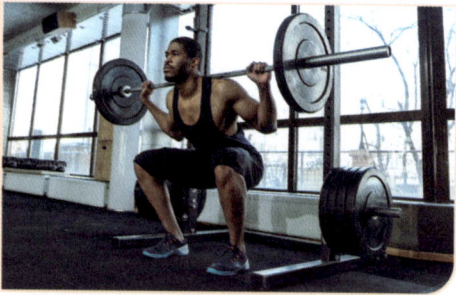

The 1RM test could be used to measure the strength of various muscle groups such as the quadriceps, latissimus dorsi, pectorals or biceps using different lifting techniques.

---

4. It is important that sports performers develop good strength. Discuss this statement. [6]

4. Strength is the ability of the muscles to exert a force.[✓] However, there are different types of strength[✓] that are useful in different sporting movements.[✓] Maximal strength is the absolute maximum force that can be generated in one muscle contraction.[✓] Static strength is the ability to hold a body part or limb in a still position,[✓] such as a handstand in gymnastics.[✓]

Dynamic strength is the ability to apply force when the muscles are continually contracting and extending.[✓] Explosive strength (power) is the product of strength and speed, i.e. strength × speed,[✓] which is useful to sprinters as they drive out of the blocks.[✓] Generally, the stronger a performer, the more efficient they will be,[✓] but some performers who lack strength can compensate for it effectively through increased skill.[✓] Strength can be measured in a variety of different ways using standardised tests.[✓]

This question should be marked in accordance with the levels-based mark scheme on page 99.

Power

Power (or **explosive strength**) is the ability to exert a maximal force in as short a time as possible. It is the product of strength and speed, i.e. strength × speed. Power can be measured using the standing or vertical jump test.

Power is crucial in **sprint sports**, **boxing**, **shot put** and **volleyball** to provide bursts of power when needed. For example, to get out of the blocks first, create a final burst to the finish line, put a shot or smash a ball with strength and speed.

Vertical jump test

The vertical jump test involves a wall, a ruler or measuring tape, and some chalk to make a mark with. With flat feet, stand and reach up the wall as high as possible and record the height.

Now, jump as high as possible using your arms and legs and make a mark using chalked hands or ask an assistant to record the height. Measure the distance between the standing reach height and the jump height in centimetres.

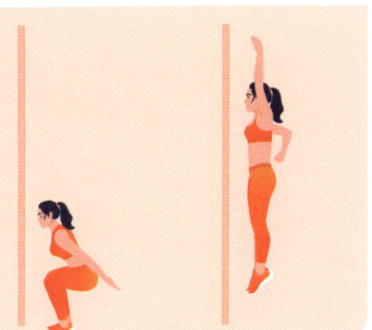

 ## Flexibility

Flexibility is a measure of the range of movement available at a joint. It can be measured using the 'sit and reach' test.

Gymnasts, **divers**, **martial artists** and **figure skaters** require excellent flexibility to increase their range of movement and to reduce injury.

Sit and reach test

Using a **sit and reach box**, the athlete sits on the floor with their bare feet flat against the box and their legs straight. The athlete then reaches forwards as far as possible to move the slider. The slider records how far in centimetres they are from zero (their feet).

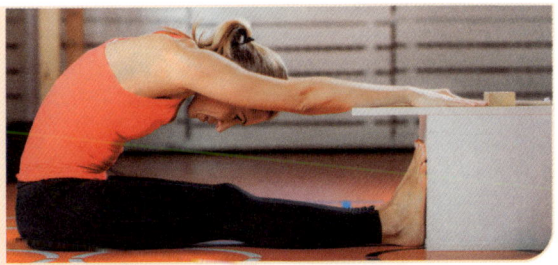

5. Give **two** reasons why a participant may not perform well on the sit and reach test. [2]

> 5. Two from: Tight hamstrings / short inelastic muscles / did not stretch or warm up,[1] injured,[1] related muscle groups are rarely used,[1] short arms and long legs,[1] males are generally less flexible,[1] the test may be measured or performed incorrectly,[1] lack of motivation to try.[1]

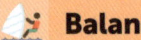 Balance

Balance is defined as the ability to stay upright or stay in control of body movement. The body's centre of mass is kept above its base. Balance can be measured using the 'stork stand' test.

Windsurfers and **horse riders** need excellent balance to continually adjust their centre of mass to stay on top of their boards and horses as they move.

Stork stand test

The stork stand test requires a **stopwatch** and an **assistant**. Time is recorded in seconds.

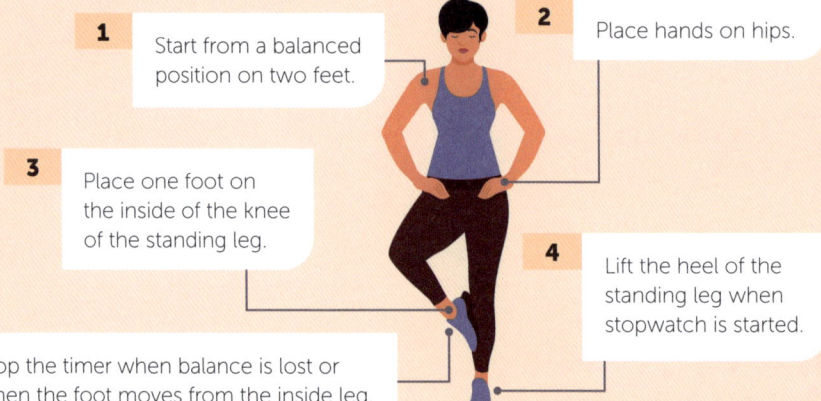

1. Start from a balanced position on two feet.
2. Place hands on hips.
3. Place one foot on the inside of the knee of the standing leg.
4. Lift the heel of the standing leg when stopwatch is started.
5. Stop the timer when balance is lost or when the foot moves from the inside leg.

Test yourself using the standard national ratings given here.

Rating	Males (seconds)	Females (seconds)
Excellent	> 50	> 30
Good	41–50	23–30
Average	31–40	16–22
Fair	20–30	10–15
Poor	< 20	< 10

6. Compare the appropriateness of the Stork Stand Test for a gymnast and a cyclist. [6]

6. The stork stand test is a maximal test. It measures static balance.[✓] The test can easily be carried out by a cyclist or gymnast as it requires no equipment / can be completed anywhere.[✓] Static strength may be used by a cyclist in a starting position or by a gymnast holding a pose.[✓] A gymnast needs excellent static balance which this measures.[✓] Gymnasts often need to balance on one leg which is also measured in this test.[✓] A cyclist requires good balance on their bike but not on their own feet[✓] and would not replicate the movements of their sport so closely[✓] so the test results may not be such a reliable measure of performance.[✓] The test could be useful to measure improvement in balance for both athletes.[✓] Overall, the test would be better for identifying strengths and weaknesses in a gymnast's balance than a cyclist's.[✓]

This question should be marked in accordance with the levels-based mark scheme on page 99.

Coordination

Coordination is the ability to move two or more body parts under control, smoothly and efficiently. It can be measured using the 'wall throw' test.

Ball and racket sports require excellent hand, eye and body coordination in order to strike the ball cleanly on a consistent basis.

Wall throw test

The **wall throw test** measures **hand-eye coordination**. It requires a **tennis ball**, a **flat wall**, some **marker tape** or **chalk**, and a **stopwatch**.

1. Mark a point or line 2 metres away from a flat wall.
2. Stand at the line with both feet together facing the wall.
3. Start the stopwatch or timer for 30 seconds.
4. Throw the ball at the wall with one hand and catch it in the other.
5. Repeat this, throwing from one hand to the other as many times as possible in the time.
6. Record the score counting each successful catch as 1.

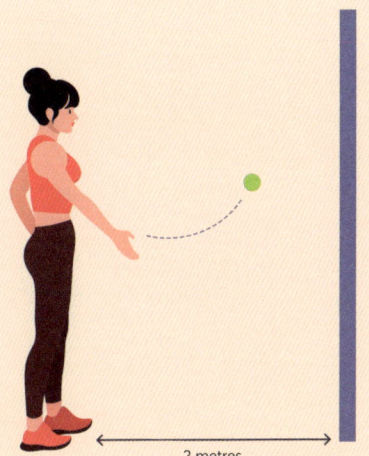

7. The table below shows the standard ratings for the wall throw test.

Rating	Excellent	Good	Average	Fair	Poor
Score (in 30 seconds)	> 35	30–35	20–29	15–19	< 15

(a) Joel scored 22. What was his rating? [2]
(b) Dominic scored 33. Compare the differences between Joel and Dominic's scores. [2]

(a) Average.[1]

(b) Dominic's score was 'Excellent' compared to 'Average'.[1] Dominic scored 11 points higher so showed better coordination.[1] Dominic may have been more motivated to do well / practised the test.[1]

OCR GCSE **Physical Education** – Topic 1.2

Reaction time

Reaction time is the ability to respond quickly to a stimulus. It can be measured using the ruler test.

Sprint racers need to react to a starting gun quickly. **Boxers** need to avoid punches.

Ruler test

Requirements: A **metre rule** and an **assistant**.

1. The assistant holds the metre rule vertically at the zero end.
2. The participant places their thumb and forefingers around the stick at the 50cm mark but without touching it.
3. The stick is released by the assistant without warning.
4. The participant must close their fingers around the stick as fast as possible to catch it.
5. The score is the distance in centimetres from the catching point to the original 50cm mark.

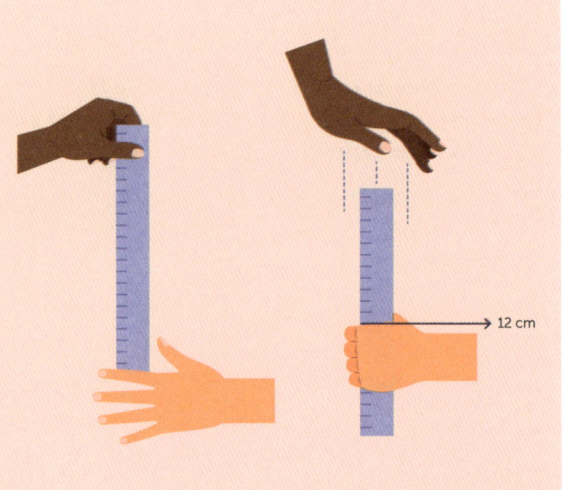

8. Figure 1 shows the ruler test reaction scores for three athletes in training over a 10 week period. Using the information in Figure 1, analyse the athlete's performance and progress. [3]

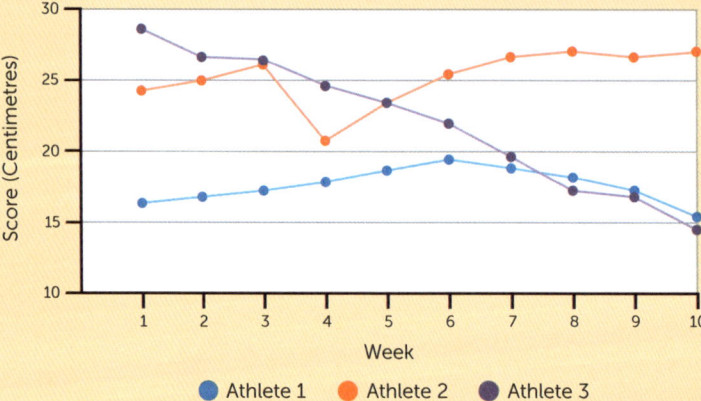

Figure 1

8. Athlete 1 had the fastest reaction time but got worse over the first five tests until they started to improve again after six weeks.[1] Athlete 2 showed relatively little change over the period but had a significant improvement in the middle.[1] Athlete 3 started relatively poorly but made the most progress with the fastest score of the three by week 10.[1]

1.2.b

THE PRINCIPLES OF TRAINING

The key principles of training use the mnemonic, SPOR.

Key principles of training

The key principles of training are provided as guidance when designing a training programme. Following the principles of training will help to make training effective. **SPOR** includes:

S   Specificity

Training programmes developed to specifically link to your training goals, sport or energy systems. For example, to build specific muscle groups identified as needing improvement, or developing specific skills related to an athlete's sport such as free kicks, set pieces in field sports or finishing in track sports.

P   Progression

Progression means to gradually increase the intensity of training so that fitness gains occur. Progress should be gradual in order to avoid injury. Progression is related to overload.

O   Overload

Overload is required to push your body beyond its comfortable limits to provide challenge, overcome plateaus and drive progress. Working harder than normal and putting your body under stress will result in adaptations and improvements to your body.

R   Reversibility

Reversibility states that athletes will undo their progress if their training schedule lapses or becomes less demanding. Fitness gains and skill levels may decrease.

The elements of FITT

The elements of FITT are useful in optimising a training plan in order to achieve fitness goals. FITT can also be used to apply the principle of overload to training. **FITT** includes:

F   Frequency

How often do training sessions happen? Two or three times a week is considered a good start but this may increase as required.

I   Intensity

How hard are the training sessions? Weights may be increased, resistance on a rowing machine may be increased or an incline may be introduced for runners.

T   Time

How long do sessions last for? As fitness increases, sessions, reps or sets may increase. Rest periods may also decrease.

T   Type

What type of training is done in each session? Switching between types of training (**pages 38-42**) adds variety, helps with overload, provides different fitness benefits and prevents boredom.

> Time out through injury is the most common cause of reversibility.

Samira is training for basketball match. How can Samira use the training principles of specificity and overload to improve her performance in the game?   [2]

Specificity: Work on the muscles / movement / energy systems used in basketball.[1] Work on agility with a ball to replicate the movements in a game.[1] Increase standing jump performance by working on the legs.[1] Practice set pieces / drills.[1]

Overload: Increase the intensity of her training workouts to challenge her maximum output.[1] Increase the regularity of training.[1] Increase the duration of her workouts.[1]

1.2.b

TYPES OF TRAINING

There are many different types of training, each with their own distinctions. Varying the type of training used helps to reduce boredom, increase commitment to fitness and avoids injury through repetitive strain.

Continuous training

Continuous training involves sustained exercise at a **constant rate** (or **steady state**) with **no rest**. It involves **aerobic demand** for a minimum of 20 minutes, for example running, swimming, rowing or cycling. Continuous training can be at any intensity.

Any training and practice method must take account of the purpose, the effects on the body and the recovery.

Advantages
- Improves cardiovascular and muscular endurance.
- Increases muscular strength in active muscles.
- Less intense on joints compared with other training methods.
- Can change body shape over time to become an ectomorph / more streamlined.

Disadvantages
- Continuous movements may result in injury from repetitive contractions.
- May not increase power as it is not anaerobic.
- Can result in tedium / boredom.
- Longer training sessions can take a lot of time.

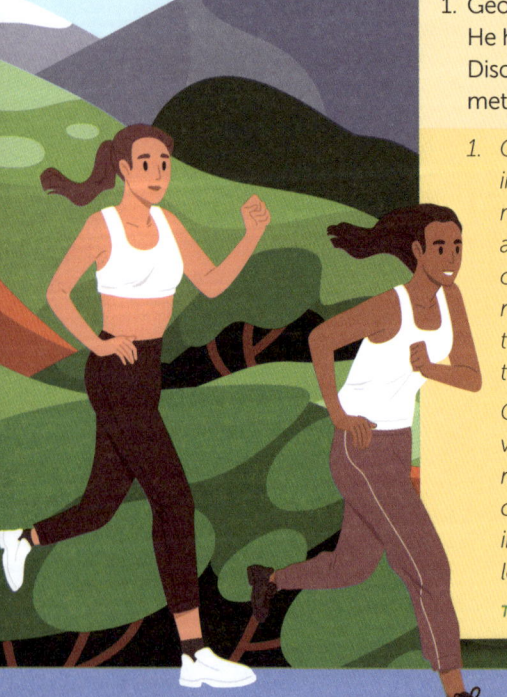

1. George is training for a marathon.
   He has chosen to use continuous training.
   Discuss whether continuous training is an effective training method for George. [6]

   1. George has chosen a form of training that has a relatively low impact on his joints and ligaments.[✓] Continuous training by running can closely replicate the movements of a marathon[✓] and requires no specialist equipment.[✓] He is likely to improve his cardiovascular endurance and may improve his body shape,[✓] reducing his weight[✓] and increasing speed.[✓] Continuous training is suitable for individuals as programmes need to be tailored which may suit George.[✓]

      George may become bored[✓] by running constantly so could vary exercise with cycling or swimming.[✓] However, this would not replicate the movements of a marathon so closely.[✓] George could supplement his training[✓] with other techniques such as interval training and static stretching to increase strength and lengthen his stride / range of motion.[✓]

      This question should be marked in accordance with the levels-based mark scheme on page 99.

Fartlek training

Fartlek is the Swedish term for 'speed play'. This involves **varying the speed**, **terrain** and **work:recovery ratios** of exercises. It is related to continuous training and interval training. Intensity is varied over different terrain, gradients or speed of activity.

Advantages

- Improves speed, cardiovascular and muscular endurance.
- Combines aerobic and anaerobic activity.
- Helps with pace and an awareness of your physical response to changes in intensity.

Disadvantages

- Needs to be tailored to the individual so unsuitable for groups.
- Requires discipline to continuously undertake unstructured exercise.
- Experience is required to ensure that training is at the right level of intensity.

2. Jo plays competitive rugby and is looking to improve her performance. Evaluate the appropriateness of Fartlek training for Jo. [6]

2. Fartlek training is known as speed play.[✓] It generally involves running and changing the speed and terrain at different points in the run.[✓] Fartlek training is ideal for game sports that consist of short bursts of anaerobic sprinting mixed with aerobic recovery periods[✓] as it helps the body to cope with varying intensities of match play.[✓] It helps to develop the use of power and explosive strength which are needed during fast game play such as a sprint to the try line.[✓] Lower intensity training improves cardiovascular endurance[✓] which is necessary to get through a match without tiring at the end.[✓] Mind/body awareness can also be improved which helps Jo understand how her body may react to sudden changes in the demand she puts on it.[✓] Jo may not be able to train using Fartlek with the whole team as the programme needs to be tailored to the individual which will differ according to their goals or player position.[✓] This may reduce the opportunity for team bonding[✓] and doesn't replicate true match conditions or gameplay.[✓] Training may improve power which will assist Jo with scrums, sprints and tackles.[✓] Since Fartlek is often used during the playing season, injury during training may mean that she misses future fixtures.[✓] Jo can use SPOR and FITT for safe and effective training.[✓] Jo may combine her training with weight training, HIIT training or plyometrics to improve all-round power and strength.[✓] Stretching and ice baths after training may help reduce delayed onset muscle soreness and improve Jo's recovery time.[✓] A change in dietary supplements to increase carbohydrates before training can also help Jo's muscles keep going in training and to repair more quickly.[✓]

This question should be marked in accordance with the levels-based mark scheme on page 99.

INTERVAL TRAINING

Interval training involves periods of exercising hard, interspersed with periods of rest or low intensity exercise. There are various types of interval training.

Circuit training

Circuit training involves roughly 6–12 **stations**, each with a different exercise designed to achieve the aims of the participants. Station activities will depend on the **space** and **equipment** available. The demand of a circuit can be altered according to the exercise or by changing the **work:rest ratio** to decrease rest and achieve overload more quickly.

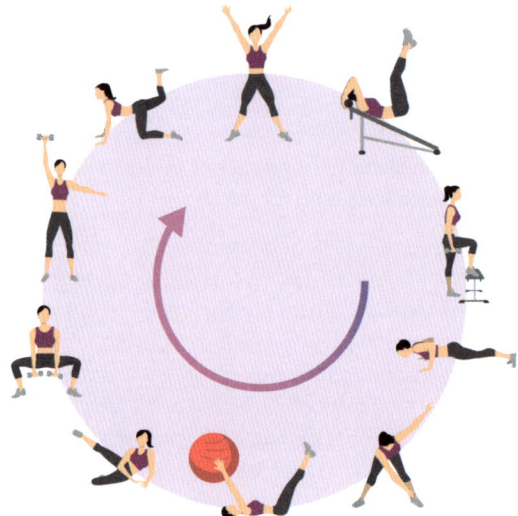

Advantages

- Can be used by large groups.
- Easy to set up.
- Usually involves little equipment so it is inexpensive to organise.
- Content or demand can be widely adapted to suit most training goals / components of fitness.
- Can be tailored to train the whole body or specific parts of it.
- Different intensities can be programmed to train aerobically and anaerobically.
- Exercises can replicate specific sporting movements

Disadvantages

- Isolated exercises may not always be totally sport specific.
- Does not replicate 'real time' match play situations or competition.
- Technique can be affected by muscle fatigue which can increase the risk of injury.

1. State what is meant by the work:rest ratio. [1]

   The period of time spent exercising at a station compared to the period of rest in between stations.

Weight training

Weight training involves lifting weights using different muscle groups to develop **strength** and **muscular endurance**. The choice of weight or exercise depends on the fitness aim. Weights may include free weights, medicine balls or resistance machines. A safe lifting technique, using a straight back, is necessary to reduce injury. A spotter may also be required to ensure safety with free weights.

Advantages
- Exercises and reps are easily adapted for specific muscular strength or endurance.
- Can be done by anyone, using anything with resistance.

Disadvantages
- Poor technique and lifting too much can cause injury.
- Muscle ache a day or so after training / DOMS is common.

---

2. Erik is a weight lifter.
   Explain how Erik can use weight training to improve maximal strength in his quadriceps. [2]

   Weights of almost the maximum weight that Erik can lift should be lifted a very low number of repetitions before resting.[1] He should repeat this for a few sets[1] with a short period of rest in between.[1]

Plyometric training

Plyometric training involves **hopping**, **bounding** or **jumping** to develop **power**, **speed** and **explosive strength**. Plyometrics makes use of gravity to extend muscles (eccentric contraction) before making a larger concentric contraction. For example, jumping off a box into a deep squat to lengthen the quadriceps before jumping higher onto another box.

Advantages
- Simulates many sporting movements such as those in high jump, volleyball, sprint starts and javelin throwing.
- No specialist equipment required.

Disadvantages
- Requires a high level of fitness to start with as there is a high risk of injury.
- Repetitive jumping and bounding can cause stress on the joints.

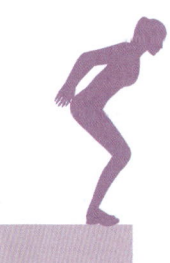

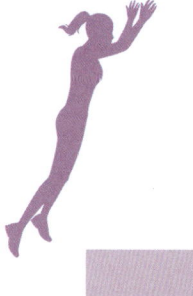

High intensity interval training

High intensity interval training (**HIIT**) increases the level of demand over standard interval training and involves more active rest. It involves the repetition of short burst of anaerobic activity.

Advantages

- Develops aerobic and anaerobic fitness.
- Easily adapted for specific outcomes and fitness components.

Disadvantages

- Can be very tiring which requires discipline and motivation.
- Intensity can cause injury if not properly managed.

---

3. Matt is a hockey player.
   Explain how interval training could be used to improve Matt's hockey performance. [2]

   Training would use sprints / anaerobic bursts[1] interspersed with rests[1] which would mimic the demands / be specific to hockey[1] as performance is at different intensities.[1]

   Hockey involves short bursts of high intensity movement / action[1] followed by active rest in slower parts of the game.[1]

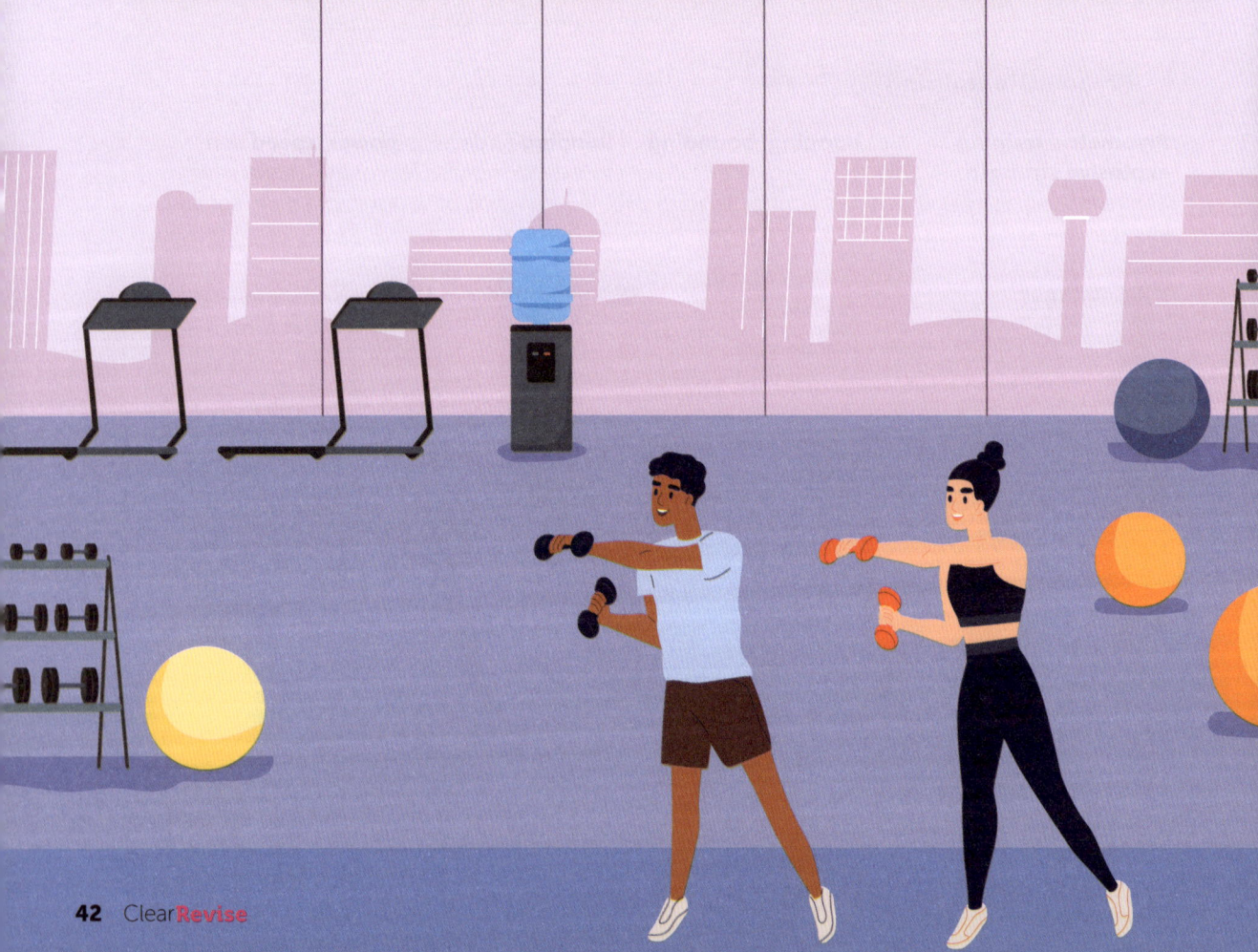

1.2.b

THE KEY COMPONENTS OF A WARM UP

Warming up routines significantly increase an athlete's ability to train to a higher level, to train more frequently, to avoid injury and to achieve better results.

Warming up

Warming up should include an activity that gradually raises the pulse, ready for exercise. Stretching the muscles increases pliability and flexibility, and reduces the risk of injury. Sports related skills and drills are also commonly included.

Physical benefits of a warm up

Pulse raising

- Warms up muscles prepares the body for physical activity
- Raises body temperature slowly
- Gradually raises heart rate up to full pace to avoid physical or mental shock

Stretching, mobility and dynamic movements

Mobility takes joints through their full range of movement in order to loosen them, for example shoulder rotations, lunges and lateral rotations of the neck. **Dynamic movements** involve speed or changes of direction.

- Improves the flexibility of muscles and joints
- Improves the pliability of ligaments and tendons
- Increases blood flow and oxygen to the working muscles
- Increases the speed of muscle contraction

Skill rehearsal

- Aids psychological preparation and confidence
- Accesses muscle memory
- Practices core or common skills, for example, a tennis player may practice serves, volleys, back hands and forehand shots.

> Dynamic movements are a key component of a warm up. Describe **two** different practical examples of dynamic exercises which could be used as part of a warm up for a named sporting activity. [2]
>
> *Shuttle runs would be helpful to a football player / tennis player to help them increase their speed and agility.[1] Skipping helps to increase speed for a boxer.[1] Zig-zagging around cones helps rugby players with side stepping.[1] High knee kicks would help a footballer or high jumper to warm up and stretch the hamstrings.[1]*

THE KEY COMPONENTS OF A COOL DOWN

Cool down routines generally involve some light activity and stretching.

Cooling down

Cooling down requires maintaining an elevated breathing and heart rate by including a walk or jog, for example. Stretching allows muscles to lengthen whilst warm, and then to relax.

A gradual reduction in intensity prevents overheating, light-headedness and nausea. It also provides an opportunity to increase post exercise oxygen consumption to repay the oxygen debt, and encourages blood flow to return to the inactive organs and away from active muscles to prevent blood pooling.

Physical benefits of a cool down

Low intensity exercise

- Helps the body's transition back to a resting state
- Gradually lowers heart rate
- Gradually lowers muscle and body temperature
- Circulates blood and oxygen back to the major organs
- Gradually reduces breathing rate
- Increases removal of waste products from the muscles such as lactic acid

Stretching

- Reduces the risk of muscle soreness and stiffness

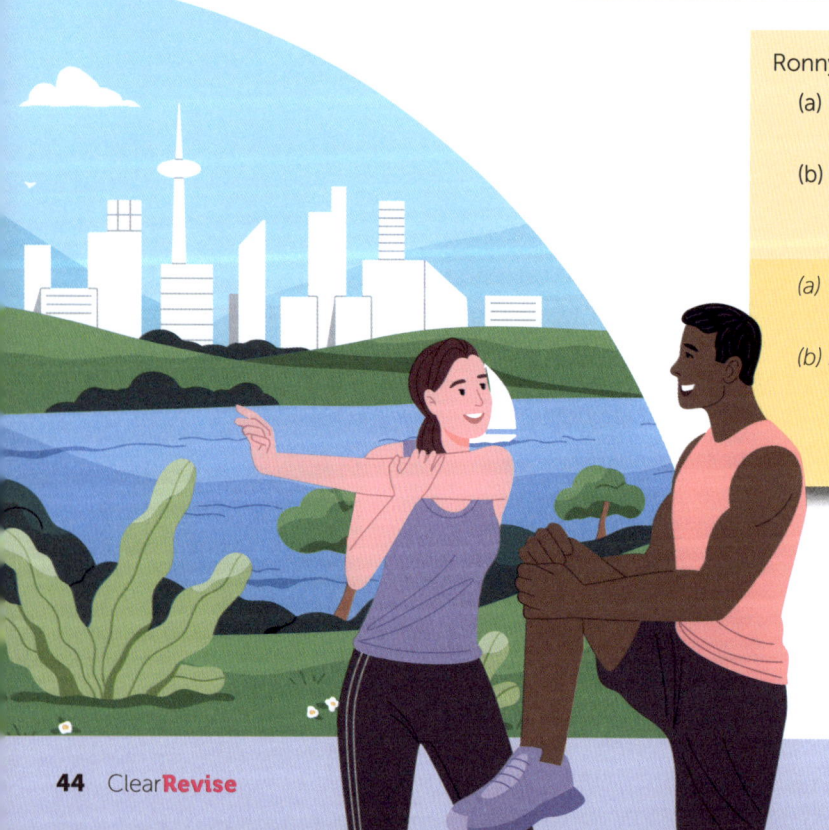

Ronny plays football for his local team.
(a) Give **one** way that Ronny could cool down after a match. [1]
(b) Describe **one** cardiovascular benefit for Ronny of cooling down. [2]

(a) Stretching,[1] gentle jog / low intensity movements.[1]
(b) Answers may include: Gradually reduces heart rate,[1] maintains circulation of blood / oxygen,[1] reduces risk of blood pooling.[1]

PREVENTING INJURY IN PHYSICAL ACTIVITY AND TRAINING

In order to prevent injury, risks can be minimised by using appropriate clothing, equipment, correct lifting techniques, using a warm up and cool down and an appropriate level of competition.

Factors in the prevention of injury

Personal protective equipment

Protective equipment, for example, a scrum cap, helmet, shin pads, gloves or gum shields can protect against injury and allow safe movement.

Correct clothing and footwear

Clothing and accessories should be appropriately sized, tied and attached. Loose clothing can cause entanglement. Loose laces could cause tripping, jewellery should be removed where applicable and hair should be tied back.

Correct footwear helps to prevent blisters, provides toe protection, ankle support and cushioning. Studs and spikes in footwear can be worn to reduce slipping.

Appropriate level of competition

Competing above your level can result in fatigue and injury. Training or activity intensity should always be matched to the individual so that it is challenging but manageable.

Lifting and carrying equipment safely

Poor technique, in lifting and throwing for example, can put too much strain on related muscles or cause other body parts to compensate unnecessarily. Contact sports (or tackling) also require the correct technique to avoid injury to either player involved. Lifting heavy sports equipment should involve at least two people, bending at the knee and keeping a straight back.

Use of warm up and cool down

Warm ups gradually increase the blood flow going to the working muscles, increasing temperature and flexibility. Warm ups also raise the heart rate in preparation for exercise.

Cooling down after exercise with a few minutes of **light physical activity** helps to maintain an **elevated breathing rate** and heart rate (**blood flow**). This eases the body out of exercise and provides continued blood flow and increased oxygen to the active muscles, which helps with the **removal of lactic acid**. See page 44.

Give **two** ways in which performers are grouped to avoid injury. Suggest a relevant sport for each. [4]

Performers are often separated by age group (youth athletics),[1] experience/skill level (skiing),[1] weight (boxing),[1] ranking (judo)[1] or gender (sprinting)[1] to help match like for like performers.[1]

1.2.c

HAZARDS IN SPORT SETTINGS

There are many hazards that need to be considered in various sports settings.

Hazard areas

Sports halls and fitness centres

- Obstructed fire exits, locked doors and windows.
- Rough wall surfaces or wall mounted fittings that could catch clothing or skin.
- Poorly lit sports areas.
- Dirty, wet, damaged or uneven flooring.
- Equipment, bags and clothing left in the way causing trip hazards.
- Poorly maintained or damaged equipment.
- Overcrowding.
- Lack of coaching and supervision can result in poor technique and irresponsible behaviour.
- Inappropriate clothing and footwear for sporting activities.

Artificial outdoor areas (e.g. Astroturf)

- Wrinkled, bald, or damaged surface can cause tripping or other injury.
- Inadequate water or sand applied.
- Poorly maintained or damaged equipment.
- Insufficient run-out space from boundary or equipment stores.
- Litter and debris, including cans, glass or stones.

Playing field

- Poorly maintained or uneven ground (e.g. with rabbit holes or mole hills).
- Badly maintained, unsecured or unsafe equipment, such as goal posts, nets and benches.
- Litter and debris, including cans, glass or stones.

Swimming pool

- Slippery, wet or damaged floor surfaces can cause a fall or cut feet.
- Loose fittings or equipment causing an obstruction.
- Overcrowding in and around the pool.
- Dirty, or poor quality water with unsafe levels of pool chemicals.
- Lack of, or inattentive lifeguards can reduce safety and encourage irresponsible behaviour.
- Deep water, or shallow areas that could cause a diving injury.

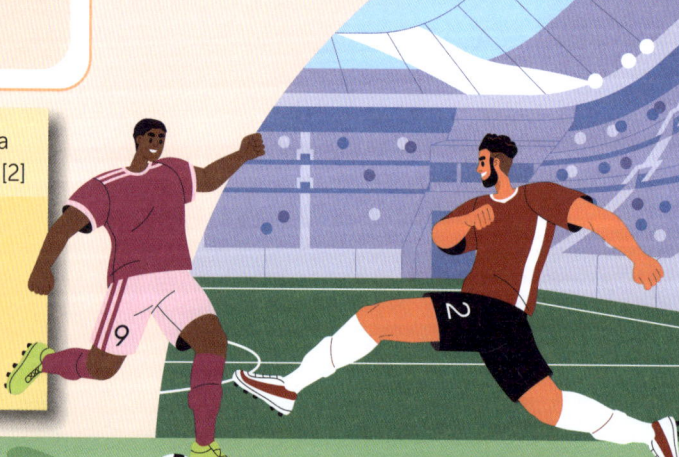

> Explain how a lack of supervision could cause a safety hazard in a sports hall or fitness centre. [2]
>
> *No one to advise on technique which could cause an injury.[1] No one to maintain any code of conduct to ensure that behaviour is good from everyone.[1] No one to manage overcrowding of rooms / equipment / stations.[1]*

46 ClearRevise

Topic 1.2

EXAMINATION PRACTICE

1. Which **one** of the following is not a component of fitness? [1]
   - ☐ A – Agility
   - ☐ B – Balance
   - ☐ C – Coordination
   - ☐ D – Decision making

2. In which of these sporting activities is reaction time most important? [1]
   - ☐ A – Lawn bowls
   - ☐ B – Motor racing
   - ☐ C – Snooker
   - ☐ D – Target shooting

3. A cricket player changes their training programme to train three times per week rather than twice a week. This is an example of changing: [1]
   - ☐ A – Frequency
   - ☐ B – Intensity
   - ☐ C – Time
   - ☐ D – Type

4. Which pair of fitness tests assess cardiovascular fitness? [1]
   - ☐ A – 30m sprint test and the press-up test
   - ☐ B – Cooper 12 minute run/walk test and the 30m sprint test
   - ☐ C – Cooper 12 minute run/walk test and the multi-stage fitness test
   - ☐ D – Sit and reach test and the multi-stage fitness test

5. Some sports performers require power.
   - (a) What is meant by 'power'? [1]
   - (b) Suggest **one** sporting activity where power would be an advantage. [1]
   - (c) Give a suitable test for power. [1]

6. Agility, balance, fast reaction time, strength and coordination are all useful components of fitness for a tennis player.
   - (a) Name **one** other component of fitness useful to a tennis player. Outline why this is important for a tennis player. [2]
   - (b) Define coordination. Discuss the importance of coordination for a tennis player. [3]

7. David and Elizabeth have been taking the Illinois Agility Test as part of their hockey club training. They are both 16 years old. David's time was 17.1 seconds. Elizabeth's time was 17.2 seconds. Analyse the data in table 1. What does it show about David and Elizabeth's performance and level of agility? [3]

Performance category	Males aged 16–19 (sec)	Females aged 16–19 (sec)
Excellent	< 15.2	< 17.0
Good	15.2–16.1	17.0–17.9
Average	16.2–18.1	18.0–21.7
Fair	18.2–18.3	21.8–23.0
Poor	> 18.3	> 23.0

National standards for the Illinois Agility Test

8. An outdoor activity centre offers rock climbing and kayaking. They have competitive teams for both sports that compete against people from other centres.

    The centre trainer has decided to use a handgrip dynamometer test to measure the strength of competitors in both sports.
    (a) Describe how to carry out this test. [3]
    (b) Evaluate whether the test is more relevant to a rock climber or a kayaker. [6]

9. SPOR and FITT are two related training principles.
    Explain how the elements of FITT can be applied to SPOR. [3]

10. Callum is a 16-year-old football player representing his local team. He warms up well using stretching techniques and has read that plyometric training could be used to improve his performance.
    (a) Give **three** factors other than stretching and warm-ups that Callum can use to help prevent injury in match play and training. [3]
    (b) Discuss the appropriateness of plyometric training for Callum and any other factors he might consider to improve his performance. [6]

11. Warming up mentally prepares an athlete for a period of intense fitness and skills training.
    Explain the physical effect on the body of warming up before training or exercise. [2]

12. Sam is responsible for safety at a training centre.
    Complete the table by identifying an example and potential injuries. [3]

Factor in injury prevention	Examples	Potential injuries
Lifting and carrying equipment safely	Poor technique	(i)
Personal protective equipment	(ii)	(iii)

TOPICS FOR PAPER 2
Socio-cultural issues and sports psychology

Information about Component 2

Mandatory written exam: 1 hour
60 marks
30% of the qualification grade
Externally assessed.

All questions are mandatory.
Use black ink. You can use an HB pencil, but only for graphs and diagrams.
Calculators are permitted in this examination.

Specification coverage

2.1 Socio-cultural influences

2.2 Sports psychology

2.3 Health, fitness and well-being.

Questions

This paper consists of a mixture of objective response and multiple-choice questions, short answers and extended response items.

2.1.a

PHYSICAL ACTIVITY AND SPORT IN THE UK

The level of physical activity and sport in the UK changes continuously, but you will need to be familiar with some general trends in participation by different social groups and in different sports.

Trends in participation in physical activity and sport

People in the UK take part in a wide range of indoor and outdoor sporting activities. The approximate popularity of different activities is shown in Figure 1. Levels of participation can be influenced by the level of funding and provision for sports in different areas of the UK.

Participation in sport can have a positive impact on mental health and well-being.

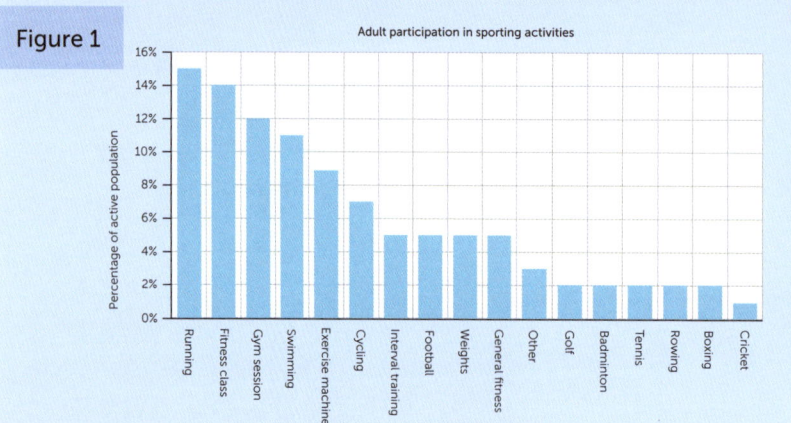

Figure 1 — Adult participation in sporting activities

Use a range of sources to find out more about participation levels in different sports. These include: Sport England, National Governing Bodies (NGBs) and the Department of Culture, Media and Sport (DCMS).

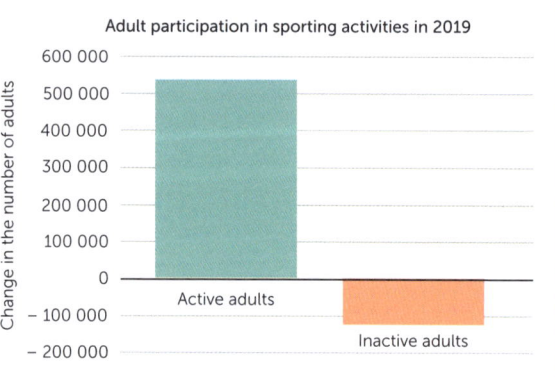

Figure 2 — Adult participation in sporting activities in 2019

In 2019, there were an estimated 28.6 million adults who regularly exercised. Participation increased by over half a million active adults from 2018.

(a) Name **one** social group contributing to a rise in adult participation. [1]

(b) The cost of living rose significantly in 2022. Explain how this impacted levels in activity. [2]

(a) Increased adult participation is primarily driven by women,[1] disabled people,[1] and those with a long-term health condition.[1] Others groups include: BAME groups, higher socio-economic groups, minority faith groups, and children and the under 21s.

(b) Those from lower socio-economic backgrounds are less likely to afford gym memberships or club fees[1] so levels of activity may decline / activity may switch to walking and jogging as it has little or no cost.[1]

50 ClearRevise

FACTORS AFFECTING PARTICIPATION IN PHYSICAL ACTIVITY AND SPORT

Different factors affect the levels of participation and engagement of different **social groups** in exercise and activity.

Social grouping by Age

Examples of factors affecting participation:

Cost

Younger people may not have the money to afford to take part in certain activities. Older people may have increased financial commitments and living costs that lower their disposable income available for activity.

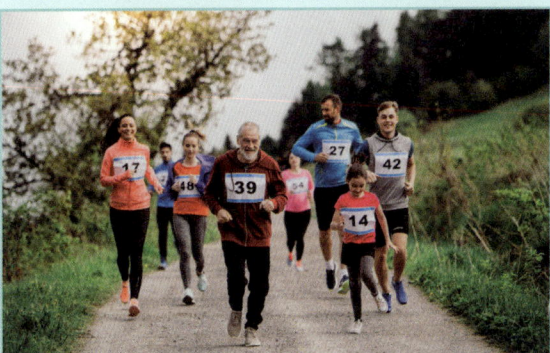

Education

Time for schoolwork may come before time for evening sports clubs. Some schools offer greater sporting provision than others. People may simply not know what is available to them.

Media coverage

An increase in media coverage of older sports performers may motivate older people to take part. Most active sports people disappear from the media when they retire which is usually only in their 30s.

Discrimination

Not all clubs and memberships are available to all **ages** - some may not allow children.

The adult participation in sporting activities for different age groups is shown in Figure 3. Give **two** reasons why the over 75s have significantly lower levels of participation. [2]

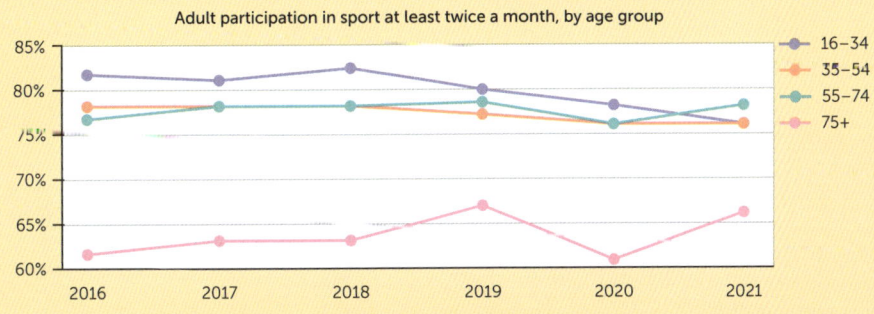

Figure 3 — Adult participation in sport at least twice a month, by age group

Answers may include: Illness / obesity / poor health,[1] poor mobility,[1] friends or social group do not participate,[1] lack of older role models,[1] self conscious / feel too old,[1] fear of injury,[1] lack of elderly sports groups / provision,[1] discrimination against the elderly.[1]

Social grouping by Gender

Examples of factors affecting participation:

Discrimination

Sexist or **stereotypical** attitudes may affect how comfortable (or not) woman feel about taking part. Most sports clubs now cater for both men and women, but some can still be largely male dominated, e.g. golf clubs.

Role models

There may be a lack of gender specific role models to inspire others of that gender to participate.

Accessibility

Regular sports teams for women may not always exist within a convenient travelling distance.

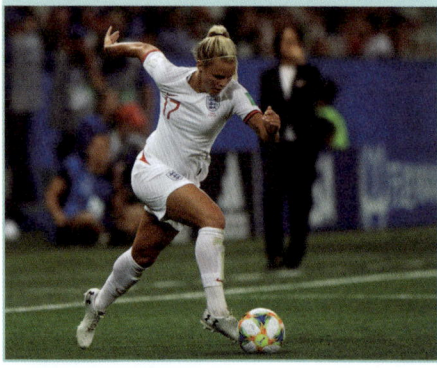

An England player during the 2019 FIFA Women's World Cup.

Media coverage

Media coverage may be more prevalent for males, compared to females.

---

1. Males are more likely to participate in sports than females. Identify **three** reasons why female participation numbers are typically below those of males. [3]
2. Calculate the percentage difference in participation between males and females. Use the data provided in Figure 4. [1]

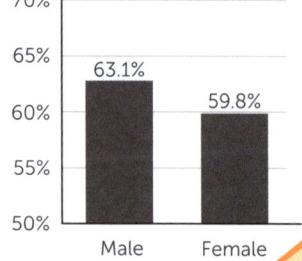

Figure 4: Sport England, November 2021.

Percentage of adults taking part in regular moderate exercise

Male: 63.1% Female: 59.8%

1. Females are less likely to take part in competitive sport.[1] Some sports are stereotypically more male oriented e.g. boxing.[1] Less funding / sponsorship available for females.[1] Discrimination / sexism in some sports.[1] Lack of female role models / less media coverage of female sports people.[1] Pregnancy / menstruation may prevent participation.[1] Childcare may be difficult to find in order to create time for sport.[1] Lack of female sports clubs / teams locally.[1]
2. 63.1 − 59.8 = 3.3%.[1]

As of 2022, the UK Chief Medical Officers' Guidelines recommend that adults should get at least 150 minutes of moderate physical activity per week. Children and young people aged 5-18 should aim to do 60 minutes of activity each day.

Moderate activity means something that raises the heart and breathing rate. This includes walking, cycling and PE classes.

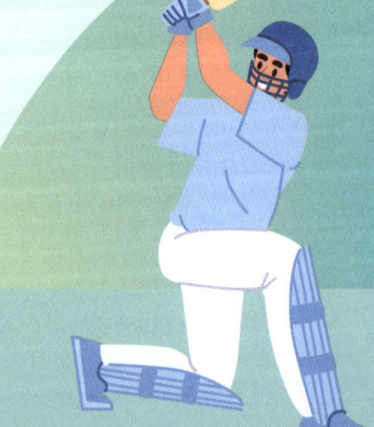

Social grouping by Ethnicity, religion and culture

Examples of factors affecting participation:

Religion and culture

Certain religions require specific clothing or commitments that may make participation harder to achieve, for example **fasting**.

Role models

There may be a lack of cultural role models for others to aspire to.

Access

It may be perceived that not all activities are inclusive for those from different cultural backgrounds.

Discrimination

Racism by other sportspeople or spectators can affect people's decision to participate in a sport, and can negatively influence a team coach's decisions. Some religious discrimination may prevent performers from wearing a hijab, or finding swimming hats to accommodate natural black hair, for example. **Homophobia** or **transphobia** may also negatively impact participation in sport.

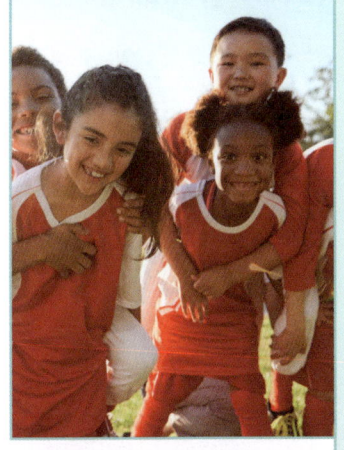

Most of the factors that affect participation can be related to any of the social groups.

For example: more media coverage, an increase in positive role models, improved education or an increase in leisure time can all positively affect the participation rates of all of the social groups.

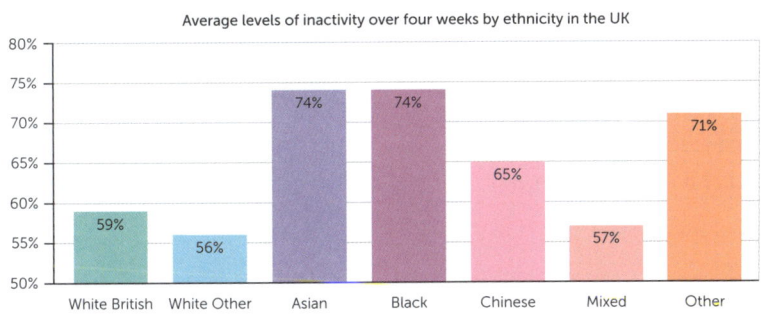

Figure 5: Sport England, November 2021

Complete the following statement using the figures and words from the box below. [3]

| highest | lowest | minority | religious | 15% | 25% |

Participation rates in sport are typically _____ by _____ groups with a difference of over _____ in the rate of participation between some groups.

Marks for: lowest,[1] minority,[1] 15%.[1]

OCR GCSE **Physical Education** – Topic 2.1

Social grouping by Family

Examples of factors affecting participation:

Role models

Active parents are more likely to have active children. They are positive role models in this respect and children will often become interested in those sports that other family members participate in.

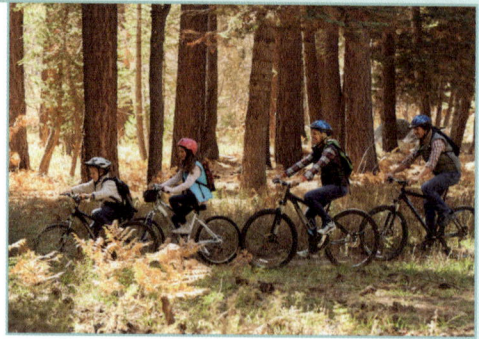

Family commitments

When adults start a family, childcare or children's activities often become a priority over their own exercise needs. This commonly reduces the amount of time for exercise in the 25–55 age groups.

Jobs often demand more time as people become more experienced or senior in their roles.

Education

Some families may not know what is available to them in their local area.

People from lower socio-economic groups are less likely to participate in regular activity than those from higher socio-economic backgrounds.

Social grouping by Disability

Examples of factors affecting participation:

Role models

There may be a lack of disabled role models to inspire disabled performers.

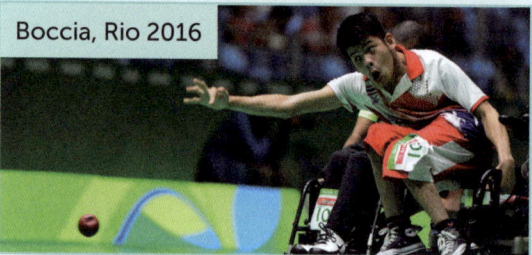

Boccia, Rio 2016

Discrimination

Some performers may feel that there is a negative **stereotype** against those with a disability.

Media coverage

Despite increased media coverage of para sports, it is still a small fraction compared to that of mainstream sports.

Access

Some facilities may not have suitable access for wheelchair users.

Participation in sport by those with a disability is around 20% lower than that of able-bodied adults.

Explain how **two** named factors can negatively affect the participation rate of people with a disability. [4]

Any two named factors with explanation: Factor: access[1] as some sports facilities do not cater for the accessibility requirements of all disabilities.[1] Factor: role models.[1] When there are only a few disabled role models, they are less able to act as an inspiration for other people with a disability to take part.[1] Factor: accessibility.[1] Some facilities may not be accessible for some disabled users.[1] Factor: stereotyping.[1] There may be a stereotype that disabled users are unable to participate.[1]

STRATEGIES TO IMPROVE PARTICIPATION

Different factors affect the levels of participation and engagement of different **social groups** in exercise and activity.

Where can you take part in boccia, polybat or squash in your area? Not sure? Perhaps there has been a lack of promotion of lesser-known sports where you live.

Promotion

People cannot participate in sporting activities that they are unaware of. Local promotion and advertising play an important part of **educating people** of the opportunities that exist around them.

Nationally, **media coverage** produces **role models** and provides inspiration for others. Promotion can encourage and influence more people to take part in physical activity by showing the benefits of regular participation.

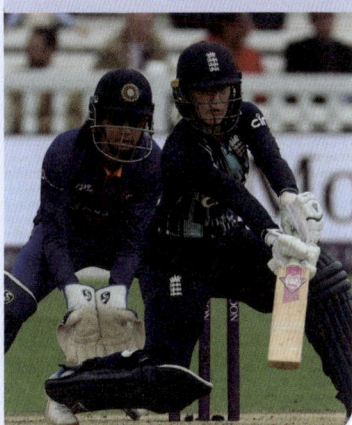

England women's cricket.

⭐ It is seldom enough in the exam to state that promotion, provision and access increase participation. The answer usually requires a reason why. E.g., "promotion can increase participation as more people are likely to want to try out an activity as awareness grows".

Provision

The right **facilities**, **equipment** and **coaching** for all groups of people need to be provided to make participation safer, easier, and at least possible. Provision is usually strongly linked to funding which can come from the media, sponsorship, local authorities or other organisations such as Sport England.

Many leisure facilities are used by schools during the day.

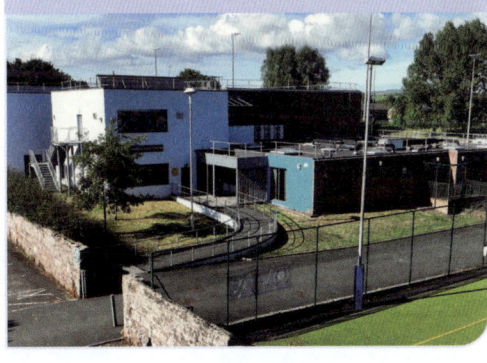

Access

Different groups have different **access requirements** which should be catered for so that everyone, regardless of age, gender, ethnicity or ability is able to have a go at some regular physical activity. Access requirements also include feeling safe, comfortable and welcome in an **inclusive environment**.

Some people can feel very self-conscious going to a fitness gym.

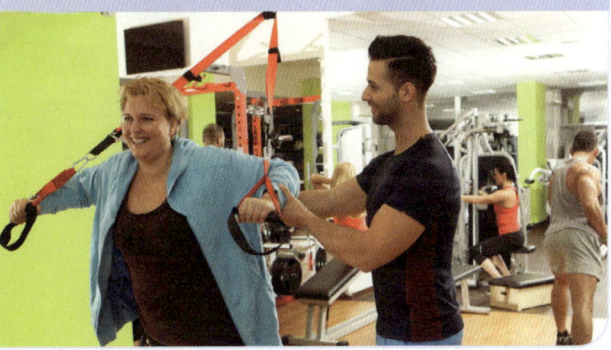

2.1.b

COMMERCIALISATION OF SPORT

Commercialisation is the influence of business on sport to make a profit which can lead to exploitation. This involves sponsorship and media coverage.

The golden triangle

The **golden triangle** is a term used to show the links and relationship between **sponsorship**, **sport** and the **media**.

Each of the three aspects in the golden triangle are reliant on each other.

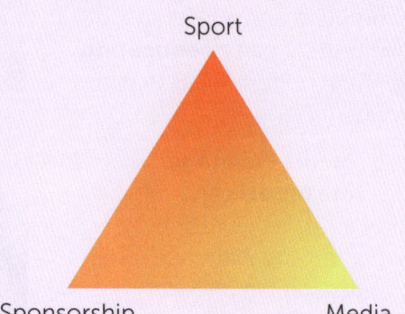

1 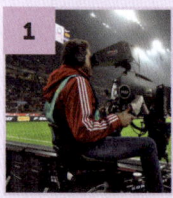 The media (usually television) pays money to the sport to be able to film and broadcast the event(s).

2 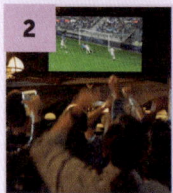 The media, for example Sky Sports, Amazon Prime or BT Sport, provides sports coverage to gain revenue from viewer subscriptions.

3 Sponsors pay money to the sport to sponsor an event.

4 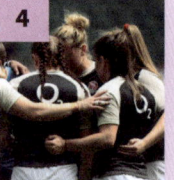 Sporting organisations receive valuable funding and income from sponsors and the media which can be invested in areas such as grass roots sport, stadia or elite athlete development.

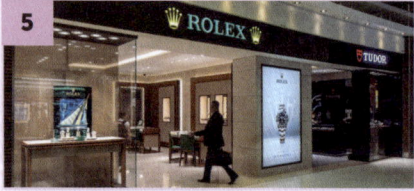

5 By sponsoring the event, sponsors increase their publicity and brand awareness which they hope will boost sales of their products and services, increasing their profit by more than the cost of sponsorship.

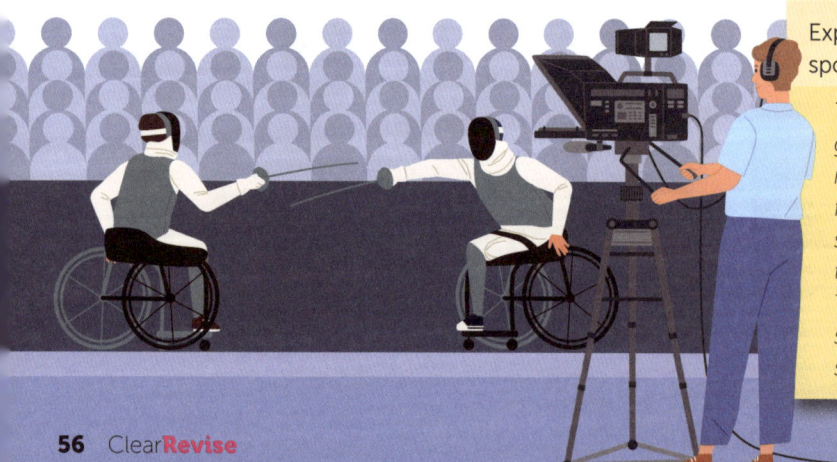

Explain the relationship between sport, media and sponsorship. [3]

The relationship is known as the golden triangle.[1] Sport receives money from sponsors and from the media.[1] Sponsors can showcase their brand to increase their profit via the media.[1] The media gain money from subscribers who want to watch the sport on television.[1]

2.1.b

TYPES OF MEDIA

The media includes social media, the Internet, TV, films, radio and other visual media, newspapers and magazines.

Media types

Social media

Social media channels include Twitter, Facebook, Snapchat, Instagram, YouTube and Strava. Advertisers can target specific groups, and users can post their own content for other users to see.

Internet

Internet media includes sports news websites, video streaming, fan sites or official club pages.

TV and visual media

TV and **film** companies pay sports bodies considerable sums for the rights to film or feature sporting action on their channels.

The channels will earn revenue by charging people to watch a film, to watch a specific feature (e.g. pay-per-view), an on-going subscription fee or, for free channels, the broadcaster will sell advertising for their revenue.

Newspapers and magazines

Newspapers and **magazines** have regular sports sections, with the back pages typically dedicated to sports. Specialist sports magazines tend to focus on single sports in greater detail. Revenue is earned through advertising revenue and print sales.

Positive effects of the media

- Quickly and effectively raises awareness of events and issues.
- Provides a good source of information, support and guidance.
- Provides entertainment and increases the appeal of sport.
- Promotes the health benefits of participation in sport.
- Encourages people, especially those in disabled or minority groups, to get more involved in activity.

Negative effects of the media

- Can be a source of incorrect information or fake news.
- Often focuses on male sports or performers in major competitions.
- Limited representation of minority groups, minor sports or para sports.
- Can highlight on-pitch errors, poor behaviour of performers and spectator trouble which detracts from the right image or reputation.
- Sports personalities featured may not be identifiable to the average person.
- Could instil a fear of failure in people through comparison of their own performances to those of elite athletes.
- May encourage watching sports rather than actual participation in physical activity.

2.1.b

SPONSORSHIP AND THE MEDIA

Sponsorship involves outside agencies or companies giving money, equipment, facilities, transport, nutritional support or scientific support to sports, sporting events or performers in return for good publicity and to increase their profit.

The positive influence of sponsorship

Sponsorship influences the commercialisation of physical activity and sport through a variety of ways:

Advantages for the sponsor

Valuable advertising for their products if they are being worn by sports stars and seen by millions.

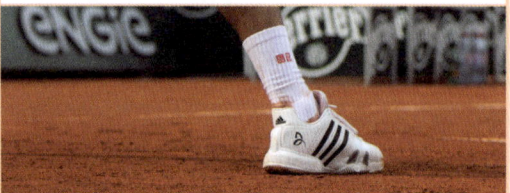

A sponsored tennis player wears Adidas.

Product or brand image is linked with success if the performer or team does well. Nike have retained their link with Michael Jordan, years after he retired.

Product association can convey aspects of sport such as success and health which may benefit sales, for example Lucozade SPORT.

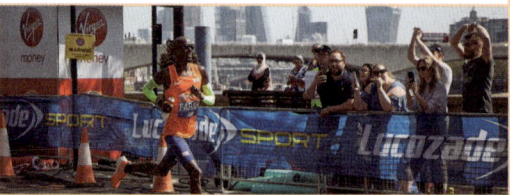

London Marathon sponsor, Lucozade Sport.

Donations to a main sports or club charity as sponsorship often benefits from tax concessions.

Merchandising and tickets sold will have a sponsor's logo attached which helps to promote their brand and strengthen any association with the sport and its relative successes.

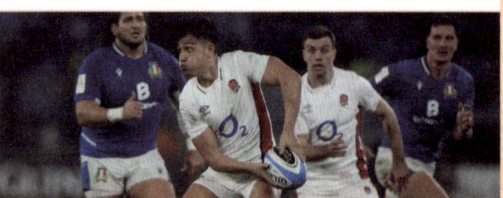

O₂ has sponsored England Rugby.

Premium tickets to their own major events are usually allocated free, to sponsors and their clients.

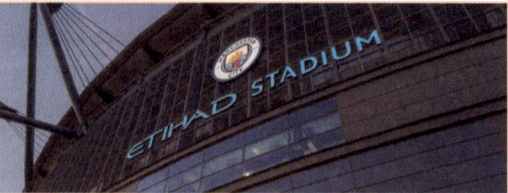

Etihad stadium of Manchester City.

The positive influence of sponsorship continued

 Sponsorship funding is necessary to provide performers with enough **money** to give up their jobs and **train full time** to enable competition at the highest levels.

 Expensive, **specialist clothing and equipment** can be paid for using sponsorship funding or donated directly by the sponsor. Wilson provides Emma Radacanu with her rackets and equipment.

 Performers can be paid substantial sums of **money** from their sponsors depending on their results. Successful athletes will be very valuable to their sponsors as their brand is reflected well through the athlete's success.

 Elite coaches can be afforded to provide the best support for performers. Sir David Brailsford is largely credited for the success of British Cycling and Team Sky.

 Medical treatment and **physiotherapy** can be paid for. Top athletes may have a full-time personal health professional. Major football clubs employ a team of health professionals dedicated to their players off and on the pitch.

 Competition or **tournament entry fees** can be very high, so sponsorship can help cover these costs. **Transport** and **accommodation** to national and global events can also be covered through sponsorship funding. British Airways provide free flights for their sponsored athletes.

 Performers may be sponsored to attend university or sports college, gaining a 'free' **education**.

 Sponsorship raises the **profile** of a performer which may enable them to increase their income through **guest appearances**, **endorsements** and **advertising**.

---

1. Using a practical example from physical activity and sport, explain **one** way in which commercialisation can have a negative impact. [2]
2. Explain how sponsorship can negatively impact a sport and its performers. [2]

1. External funding can be relied upon and withdrawn at no notice as they do not want to be associated with poor performance, injury or misbehaviour.[1] Anthony Joshua lost sponsorship when he lost his world heavyweight title.[1]

   Minority sports / groups rarely attract enough attention to engage major sponsorship as the sponsors want large audiences[1] which means these sports continue to struggle in terms of their own funding and promotion. Women's football clubs are paid only a fraction by their sponsors than men's clubs.[1]

   Some sponsorship companies may promote unhealthy drinks or foods / undesirable products or services (e.g. alcohol or gambling)[1] which may create an unwelcome association with sport. McDonalds faced a backlash after its sponsorship of the Olympics.[1]

   Accept any suitable sporting examples.

2. Sponsors can assert powerful influence over a sport in order to gain the widest audience or to accelerate the action which may not be in the best interests of its performers.[1] Sponsorship funding can apply too much pressure on performers to succeed for fear that the sponsorship would end otherwise.[1] Sponsorship commitments may distract a performer from their sport, meaning performance levels drop and they therefore risk losing the funding.[1]

2.1.c

ETHICS IN SPORT

Sport should be played in the manner it is intended. Bending or breaking the rules can have serious consequences for performers and the reputation of their sport.

Ethics is a set of moral principles based on what is deemed right and wrong, not simply what is legal or illegal.

Sportsmanship

Sportsmanship means **fair play**. It is ethical, appropriate, polite and fair behaviour while participating in a game or athletic event.

Performers who show good sportsmanship will:
- Avoid cheating, foul play or aggression.
- Be friendly to all competitors and avoid unpleasantness.
- Take measures to reduce the risk of injury to others.
- Help injured players before playing on.
- Promote their sport in a positive way and be a positive role model.
- Accept the decision of umpires, referees and officials.

Deviance

Deviance means behaviour that is either immoral or seriously breaks the rules and norms of a sport. Deviance and gamesmanship have a fine line between them, but they both tend to happen when sports people place too high a priority or importance on winning over anything else.

Deviance includes cheating, violence, taking performance enhancing drugs and match fixing.

Gamesmanship

Gamesmanship means pushing the rules to gain unfair advantage. The laws of a sport may be interpreted in ways which, whilst not illegal, are not in the spirit of the game. Coaches can also be guilty of encouraging such behaviour.

Examples of gamesmanship include:
- Football players wasting time with the ball in anticipation of the final whistle.
- Tennis players deliberately calling 'out' when the ball was 'in'.
- Runners jostling for position on the track.
- A golfer coughing to distract an opponent in a putt.
- Rugby players attempting to move the penalty spot slightly closer to the posts than where the infringement took place.
- Cricket bowlers sledging a batsman to intimidate them.

Give **one** reason for gamesmanship in sport. [1]

To increase the likelihood of winning / to turn the game around if losing.[1] To gain fame / financial reward for winning.[1] To feel clever by 'playing' the rules to their letter.[1] Copying the behaviour of others.[1] Frustration of losing a point / being in a losing position.[1] Orders from the coach.[1]

VIOLENCE IN SPORT

Violence is defined as any physical acts committed in sport that go beyond the accepted rules of play or the expected levels of contact within a contact sport.

Reasons for player violence

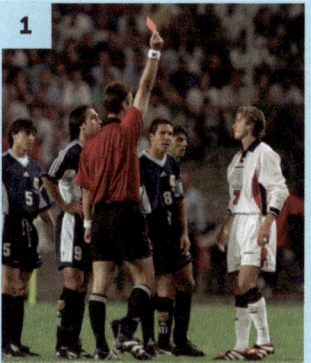

1. Instinctive response – Sometimes the moment engages a fight or flight response which is difficult to control.

In a "moment of madness", David Beckham kicked Argentine Diego Simeone during a World Cup match in 1988. He was sent off with a red card and England lost the match on penalties.

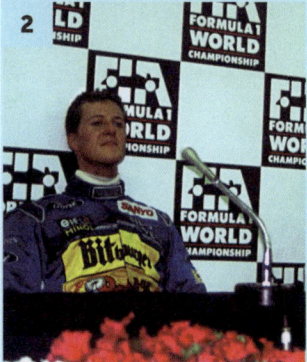

2. To enhance performance – Performers can bring down others to improve their own outcome.

Schumacher appeared to turn in aggressively against Damon Hill in the last race of the 1994 F1 Championship, ultimately putting both cars out of the race and handing himself a win by one point.

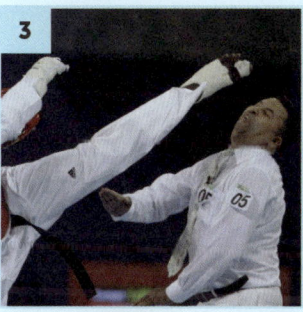

3. Frustration – Losing a match or game that players are expecting to do well in can cause performers to lose control of themselves.

Taekwondo's Angel Valodia Matos kicked a referee after being disqualified from his bronze medal bout.

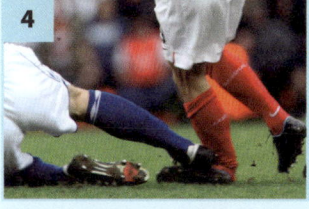

4. Copying others – Many performers copy poor technique from older colleagues.

In 2008, Taylor tackled da Silva so hard it broke his leg in four places.

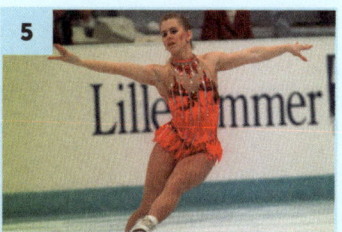

5. Pressure to win – Some performers will do anything at any cost to win.

In 1994, Tonya Harding won her ice-skating championship after her main rival was attacked with a baton, putting her out of the competition. Harding and accomplices were later convicted with related charges. Harding was banned for life.

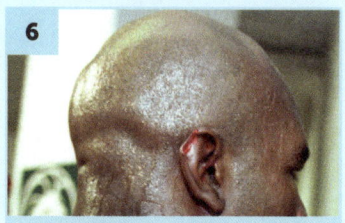

6. Retaliation, revenge or intimidation – Some performers deliberately attack others when they feel wronged.

Underdog boxer, Evander Holyfield's ear was bitten off by opponent Mike Tyson in 1997 after Holyfield dominated the early rounds of the fight.

2.1.c

DRUGS IN SPORT

In the pursuit of success, sports performers may turn to illegal drugs to enhance their performance and give themselves an unfair advantage over other competitors.

Why sports performers use drugs

Performance enhancing drugs are taken for a wide range of reasons. Many performers think they will never get caught and can get away with it. Others may be under considerable pressure from coaches to take drugs or to perform better. Further reasons include:

- To improve components of physical fitness, for example strength, speed or power.
- To reduce or mask pain.
- To increase levels of aggression.
- To reduce performance anxiety, calm their nerves and lower their heart rate.
- To build muscle mass.
- To increase their levels of arousal and alertness.

Types of drugs and their effect on performers

Anabolic steroids

Anabolic agents increase the rate and amount of muscle growth and speed up recovery time. Side effects include over-arousal, causing a negative impact on performance as well as heart damage and high blood pressure.

Beta blockers

Beta blockers help to control heart rate and reduce anxiety, keeping a performer calm. They can block adrenaline, lowering arousal and improving focus; an unfair advantage in sports that require fine motor skills such as shooting, archery and golf.

However, they can have serious side effects including nausea, poor circulation, heart problems and weakness.

Stimulants

Stimulants can increase reaction time, alertness and concentration in order to mask tiredness or fatigue, or to function better. They can also raise confidence levels and aggression, elevating performance in endurance and power sports.

Playing beyond your natural abilities can, however, increase the chance of injury. Performers can also become addicted to stimulants. They can experience insomnia and increase their risk of heart disease, high blood pressure and liver disease.

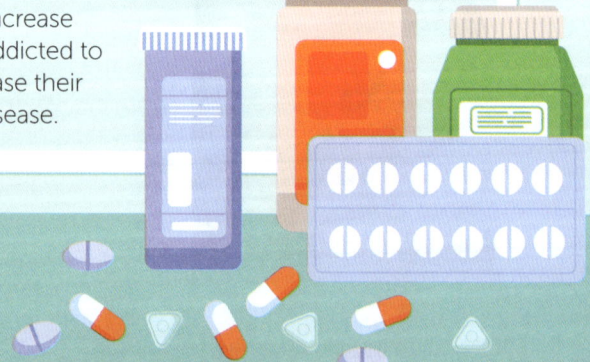

US Athlete Marion Jones admitted to taking steroids in the Sydney Olympics. She was stripped of her medals and banned from the Beijing Games.	North Korean Shooter Kim Jong-Su was expelled from the Beijing Olympic village after testing positive for beta blockers.	Romanian footballer Adrian Mutu was found to have taken stimulants so faced a nine month ban and around €17m in damages.

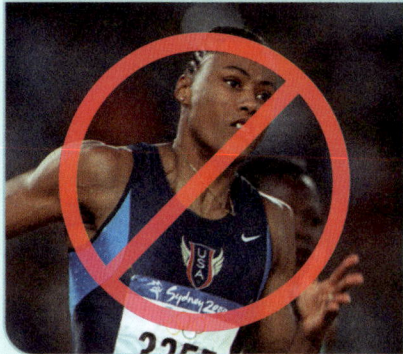 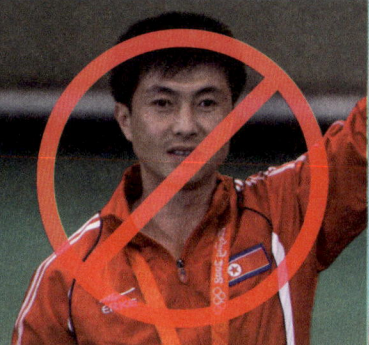 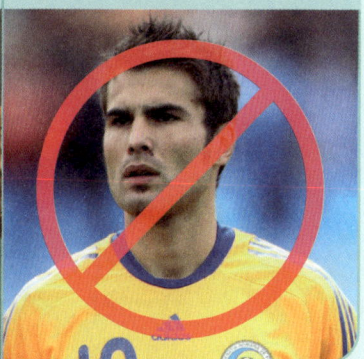

Discuss the impact of taking anabolic steroids on a sprinter and their performance. [4]

Sprinters can gain an advantage through increased muscle mass which will increase their power, allowing them to run faster.[1] Steroids increase aggression and competitiveness which is an advantage in explosive events such as the 100 metres.[1] Winning could increase a sprinter's level of fame / income / sponsorship.[1]

Being caught would irreparably damage their reputation.[1] They would likely be removed from the team.[1] They may be banned from the sport.[1] A fine is commonly imposed which they would need to pay.[1] Sponsors are likely to drop their support immediately.[1] The performer may become addicted / could suffer health problems.[1]

The impact on sport

The reputation of an entire sport or sporting body rests on the actions of individuals within it.
- The reputation of a sport could be heavily damaged if many competitors are found to be using drugs.
- The sports body could lose their key sponsorship leading to a loss of income.
- Spectator numbers and the overall fan base may decline, reducing interest, media coverage and income from ticketing and merchandise.
- Participation levels may fall if others perceive that success is only possible with performance enhancing drugs.
- People may lose trust in past and future results.
- There would need to be a difficult, awkward and embarrassing process to revisit previous results to redistribute medals and awards to fair performers.
- More funding would need to be invested into drug testing instead of helping emerging or elite athletes to perform to higher standards.
- Honest or 'clean' athletes can lose credibility if they are suspected or assumed to drug users.

Topic 2.1

EXAMINATION PRACTICE

1. Suggest why the percentage of active adults typically increases between March and October each year. [1]

2. Identify **two** social groups that have typically lower levels of participation in sport compared to the national averages. [2]

3. The charts in Figures 1 and 2 show the levels of disposable income and the levels of physical activity across the UK.

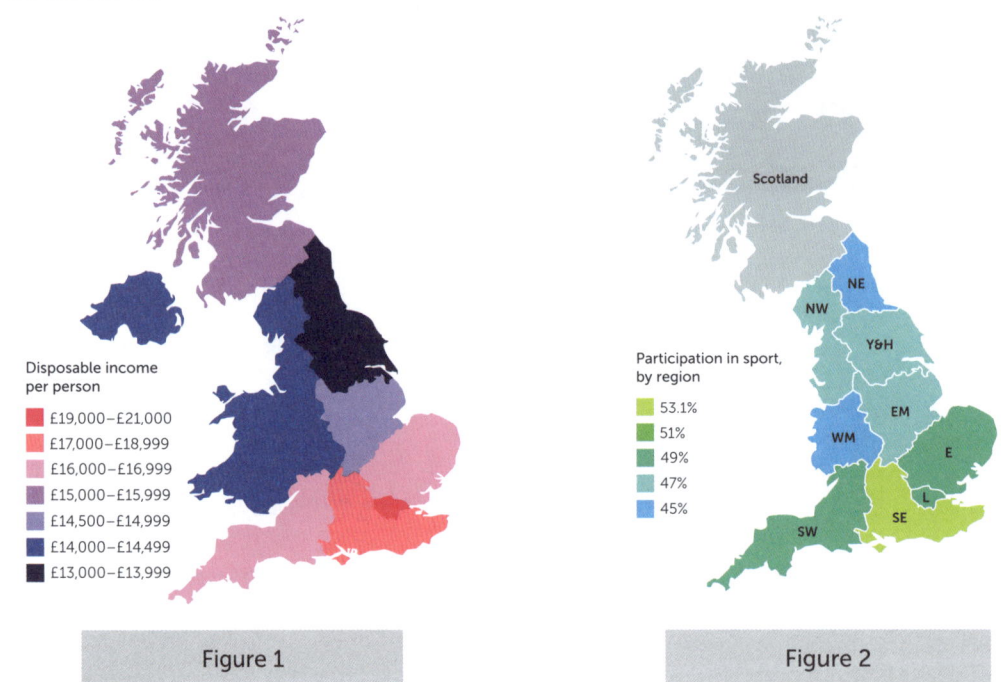

Figure 1   Figure 2

   (a) From the information provided in Figures 1 and 2, explain the relationship between disposable income and levels of activity. [1]
   (b) Estimate the level of activity in Scotland as a percentage. [1]
   (c) Calculate the percentage difference between the most and least active areas of the UK. [1]
   (d) Analyse **two** ways that local authorities can increase the level of participation in sports by adults. [6]

4. Which **one** of the following does not form part of the golden triangle? [1]
   - ☐ A – Commercialisation
   - ☐ B – Media
   - ☐ C – Sponsorship
   - ☐ D – Sport

5. Sponsorship support can come in different forms.
   (a) Complete the following definition of sponsorship using the words in the box.
       Each word chosen can only be used once. [4]

   | increase   decrease   results   publicity   money   companies   performers |

   The giving of _____ or goods to _____ in order to get good _____ and/or _____ profit.

   (b) Other than facilities, clothing and equipment, give **one** other type of sponsorship support. [1]
   (c) For **two** of the sponsorship types given below, provide a named example. [2]

   Facilities e.g. stadia: _____

   Clothing _____

   Equipment _____

6. Describe how **two** named types of media can be used to broadcast sport. [4]

7. Ethics in sport considers the elements of sportsmanship, gamesmanship and deviance.
   Draw a line from each of the elements to match the correct practical example. [2]

   Sportsmanship   Making a deliberately hard tackle to injure or intimidate another player

   Gamesmanship   Kicking a ball off the pitch if any another player is injured

   Deviance   Over-celebrating a goal to dampen the spirits of the opposition

8. Performance enhancing drugs are used in sports.
   (a) Some athletes are encouraged to take performance enhancing drugs owing to pressure from their coaches. Is this statement true or false? [1]
       ☐ True
       ☐ False
   (b) Which **one** of the following performance enhancing drugs increases muscle mass? [1]
       ☐ A – Anabolic steroids
       ☐ B – Beta blockers
       ☐ C – Diuretics
       ☐ D – Stimulants
   (c) Give **two** advantages to a boxer of taking stimulants. [2]
   (d) Discuss the impact on the sport of boxing if performers are regularly found to be taking performance enhancing drugs. [4]

9. Give **two** reasons for player violence in sport. Provide a practical example for each. [2]

2.2

CHARACTERISTICS OF SKILFUL MOVEMENT

Skilful movement is characterised by fluent and coordinated action which is efficient, technically accurate and aesthetically pleasing.

Motor skills

Motor skills are actions that involve movements of the body. They are learned and all lie on a **muscular continuum**:

Rugby tackle — Javelin throw — Golf putt
Gross skills ——— Fine skills

You can place a skill anywhere on a continua as long as you can justify it.

At one end, **gross skills** use large muscles or muscle groups to perform big, strong, powerful movements. At the other, **fine skills** are responsible for small and precise movement, requiring high levels of accuracy and coordination. Fine skills involve the use of a small group of muscles.

The characteristics of skilful movement

Efficiency

Some performers act with effortless **efficiency**, wasting very little energy in their common actions, for example hockey players passing the ball between each other.

Coordination

Many skills can be combined into a longer movement in a display of **coordination**, making sure that one action is linked with the next, and that movement involving any equipment, such as balls, rackets and approaching hurdles is synchronised.

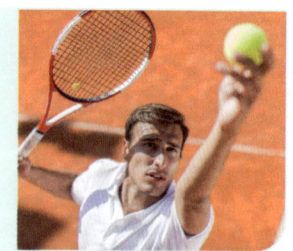

Fluency

Skills can be combined into one fluid and natural-looking movement, for example catching a ball on your foot and moving smoothly into a dribble, which turns **fluently** into a shot on goal.

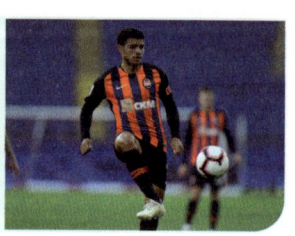

Pre-determination

Some skills have **pre-determined** movements and expected outcomes, for example, knowing where to place a rugby ball in a conversion kick, where on the court to serve a squash ball, or a predetermined ice-skating routine.

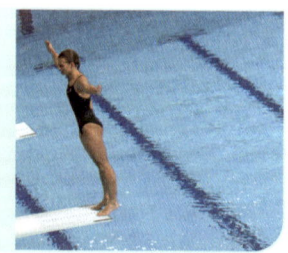

Aesthetic

An **aesthetic** skill is one that looks good when performed. A stylish and well-executed BMX or freestyle skiing trick has strong aesthetics.

2.2

CLASSIFICATION OF SKILLS

Different sports require different sets of skills for performers to acquire and perfect.

Skill and ability

A **skill** is a learned action or learned behaviour with the intention of bringing about predetermined results, with maximum certainty and minimum outlay of time and energy.

An **ability** is an inherited, stable trait that determines an individual's potential to learn or acquire a skill.

> ★ Skill classifications are continuums. A skill may lie somewhere on a line between one extreme and the other. You may need to justify why a skill is nearer one end than another.

Classifications of skill

Skills can be classified in two ways:

Difficulty continuum: Simple to complex

A **simple skill** (e.g. jogging) requires few decisions to be made that affect the skill so they are learned quickly and require a low level of coordination or concentration to complete.

A **complex skill** (e.g. batting in cricket) requires lots of decisions in order to be successful and requires a high level of coordination and concentration.

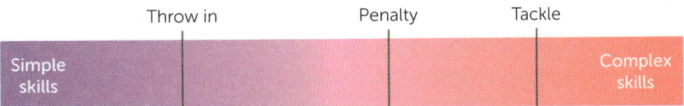

Environmental continuum: Open to closed

An **open skill** (e.g. football tackle) is performed in a certain way to deal with a changing or unstable environment, e.g. the position or movement of an opponent will affect how you should tackle them.

A **closed skill** (e.g. platform dive) is one which is not affected by the environment or performers within it. The skill tends to be done the same way each time.

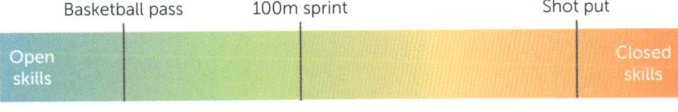

Classify the skill of bowling a cricket ball using each of the three continua. Justify each classification. [3]

Complex as it requires making decisions about the type and placement of the ball with several movements involved in the run-up and swing.[1]

Closed as it is performed the same way each time.[1] *Accept open as it may depend on the batsman's stance, condition, style and weather conditions.*[1]

Gross motor skills as it involves big movements of the arm and body.[1] */ Fine motor skills are involved by the fingers to control the ball / spin / to precisely hit the stumps.*[1]

2.2

GOAL SETTING

Sporting goals vary according to what the performer wants to achieve. Goals can be set by athletes themselves, or by their coaches.

SMART targets

SMART targets are appropriately defined goals that can be used to improve and/or **optimise performance**. They can **motivate performers** to achieve **exercise goals**, provide additional **interest** to activity, and help **adherence to training**. Goals can also **reduce stress** and **improve focus**.

S — Specific
Goals must be specific to the demands of the sport, the muscles or the movements used.

M — Measurable
It must be possible to measure whether a goal has been met.

A — Achievable
Goals should actually be possible to complete / within capability.

R — Recorded
Measurements of progress should be evidenced.

T — Time-bound
A set period of time or deadline by which the goal will be achieved.

Nina says she wants to improve her golf handicap. Identify **one** way in which she can make this goal SMART. [1]

Specific – Nina needs to state how many points she wants to reduce the handicap by / the target handicap. [1] *Achievable – Nina needs to be confident that she is capable of reaching her goal in the time given.* [1] *Recorded – Nina needs to record her golf scores for each round she plays.* [1] *Timed – Nina needs to state a date by when the goal should be met.* [1] *The goal is already measurable.*

Beginner skier

S — I will learn to link turns using parallel skis in the traverse.

M — I will ski for four hours each day, for one week.

A — My instructor and I agree that this is realistic and that I can do it

R — The goal is written down and observed by the instructor.

T — I will achieve it by the end of the week.

Downhill racer

S — Improve my start time by keeping my poles nearer my feet for a faster split in the top section.

M — I will shave off an average 0.6s from my first split time.

A — The coach says I am capable and I am getting better.

R — Goals and races times can are recorded to evidence progress against aims.

T — I will achieve it in 28 days of practice.

68 ClearRevise

2.2

MENTAL PREPARATION

Mental preparation is used by performers to rehearse a physical skill within their minds without any actual physical movement.

Mental rehearsal, visualisation or imagery

By mentally picturing themselves performing a skill perfectly and imagining positive outcomes before attempting it (such as a podium finish), sportspeople can relax and focus on their performance. These are common techniques used by performers such as long- and high-jumpers, football players before a penalty kick, or divers before leaving the platform. This gives them time to think through their technique, to form a successful strategy and to prepare themselves for the action.

Visualisation and **imagery** can also be used to imagine being in a calm, relaxing environment, blocking out the noise and pressure from a large audience for example.

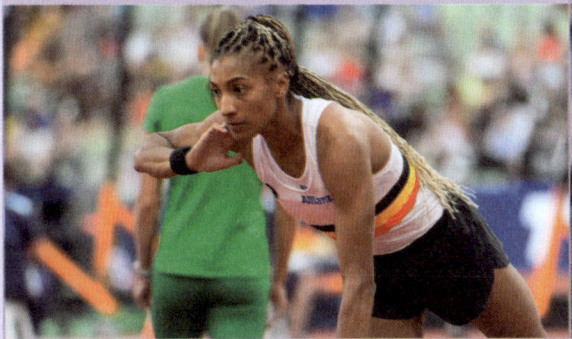

A Belgian athlete mentally rehearsing the women's heptathlon shot put.

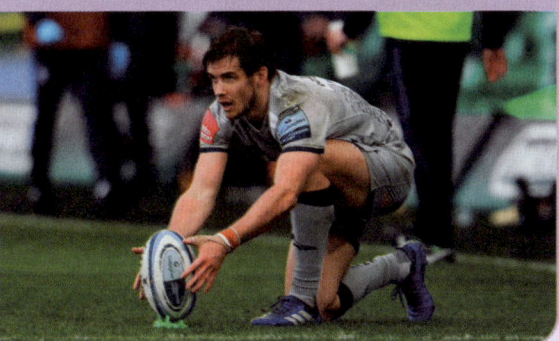

A rugby player uses visualisation and imagery before taking a conversion kick.

Positive thinking

Self-talk is a psychological technique involving the performer giving themselves instructions and words of encouragement in their head.

Selective attention

A performer will take a lot of information from their environment in the midst of the action, for example, they may see a ball being struck and coming towards them.

By focusing on the most important element of their surroundings, (e.g. the ball flying through the air and how to receive it) they block out irrelevant information (for example, the crowd). This is called **selective attention**.

> Give an example of positive thinking for a named sport of your choice [1]
>
> *Examples include: I am going to clear all of the jumps on my horse. / I am going to kick the ball between the goal posts for a rugby conversion. / I have jumped this height before so I can do it again.* [1]

OCR GCSE **Physical Education** — Topic 2.2

2.2

TYPES OF GUIDANCE

Coaches need to identify the most appropriate methods to provide guidance to beginners or elite level performers to aid the learning of a skill.

Types of guidance

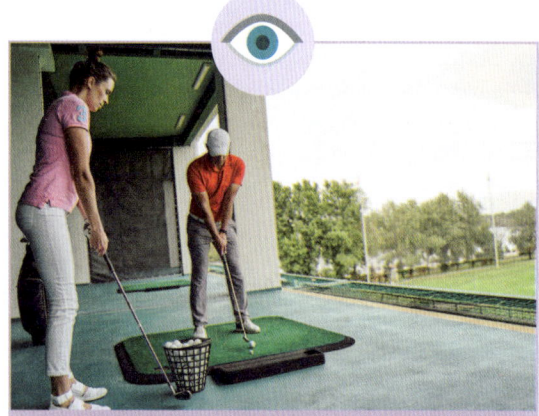

Visual (seeing)

Visual guidance involves the use of demonstrations that allow the performer to 'see' the skill. This includes watching an instructor, video, images or diagrams.

- ➕ Quick and concise which is good for beginners to create a mental picture that they can copy
- ➕ Slow motion replays can be used for detailed analysis of complex skills
- ➖ Complex skills can be difficult to demonstrate clearly
- ➖ Performers need to be paying close attention.

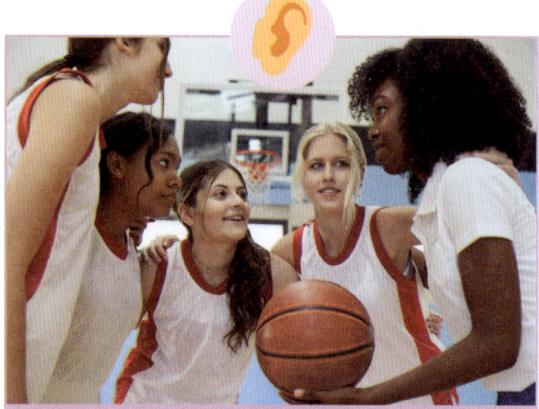

Verbal (hearing)

Coaches or instructors will provide explanations of how to do things, or audible cues on when to move or hold a position.

- ➕ Can be provided whilst a sporting action is being performed
- ➕ Easily combined with other forms of guidance
- ➖ Less suitable for beginners if technical language is used
- ➖ Complex skills are difficult to explain in words.

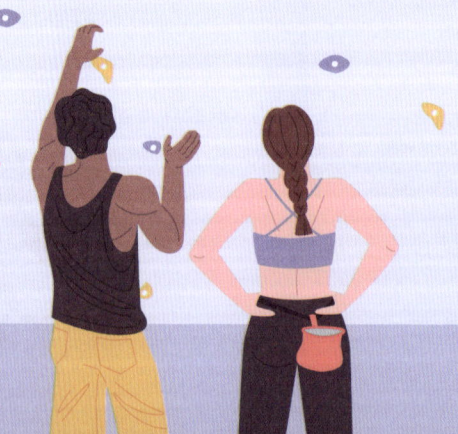

Types of guidance continued

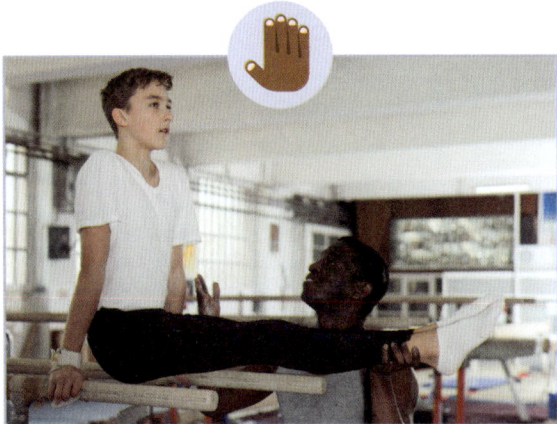

Manual (Physical assistance with movement)

Coaches may physically manipulate the athlete through the skill by moving body parts into the correct position, stance or through a complete range of motion.

- ➕ Useful for beginners to get the feel of a movement or position, or for safety
- ➕ Subtle positioning can be adjusted to develop complex skills
- ➖ Useful on an individual basis only rather than with sports teams
- ➖ Less suitable for elite performers
- ➖ Physical contact requires consent.

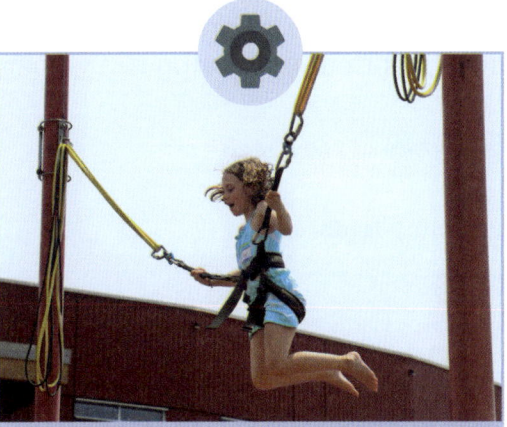

Mechanical (use of objects or aids)

Sports equipment is used to assist the performer, for example, swimming paddles, arm bands or tennis ball machines.

- ➕ Useful for beginners to 'feel' the motion, technique or for safety
- ➕ Builds confidence without the fear of injury
- ➖ Performers may come to rely on the support
- ➖ Mistakes in technique using the aids can become engrained.

State the type of guidance being provided in each example below:

(a) A child is using stabilisers to learn to ride a bike. [1]

(b) A boxer's arms are physically moved into the correct guard positions by their coach. [1]

(a) Mechanical.[1]
(b) Manual.[1]

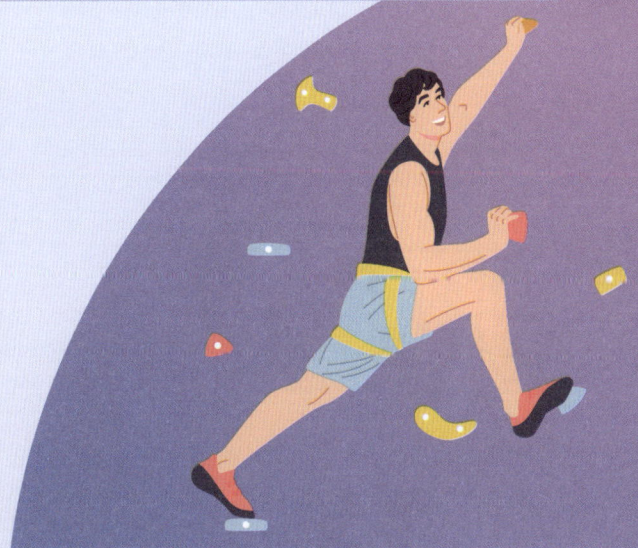

OCR GCSE **Physical Education** – Topic 2.2

2.2
TYPES OF FEEDBACK

Feedback can be given to a sportsperson either during or after their activity with the aim of improving future performances.

Types of feedback

Positive feedback – Explains what a performer is doing right, e.g. *"Excellent follow through"*.

Advantages – Essential for motivation, confidence and reassurance.

Disadvantages – Could give a false picture of actual performance.

Negative feedback – Explains what a performer is doing wrong e.g. *"Keep your chin tucked in"*.

Advantages – Commonly used to focus more efficiently on precisely what to improve

Disadvantages – Can be demoralising for beginners

Knowledge of results – Provides feedback on the outcome, for example *% first serves in, score, time or distance*.

Advantages – Useful as a quick measure of success after the event. Knowing the result builds confidence in progress.

Disadvantages – Can be an average set of results or trend provided long after the event.

Intrinsic (or **kinaesthetic**) **feedback** – comes from within. It is 'felt' by the performer through their own senses or muscles.

Advantages – Beginners do not usually have enough experience to have developed a feeling for the correct technique.

Disadvantages – Elite athletes have a strongly developed sense of their own performances that they can 'feel'.

Extrinsic feedback – Is provided by an outside observer, commonly a coach.

Advantages – Useful for beginners who are less aware of what a successful technique looks or feels like, and when they don't know how to improve.

Disadvantages – Elite performers may have to combine extrinsic and intrinsic feedback.

Knowledge of performance – Focuses on individual elements of a performance, for example, *grip, stance, start* or *follow through*.

Advantages – Helps to fine tune specific elements of a performance..

Disadvantages – Can be too detailed for beginners so it is often simplified.

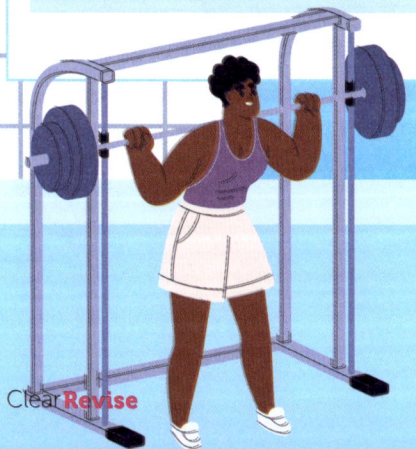

Dana is a competitive weight lifter. She uses a wall mirror when she is training to gain feedback. Explain why an athlete may use a wall mirror to gain feedback. [3]

A mirror provides an instant knowledge of performance[1] which helps to develop / fine tune technique.[1] Extrinsic feedback from the mirror[1] can help to develop / fine tune intrinsic feedback.[1]

Topic 2.2

EXAMINATION PRACTICE

1. Give **one** example of a predetermined skill and **one** example of an aesthetic skill. [2]

   Predetermined skill: _____

   Aesthetic skill: _____

2. Sports involve a range of skills.
   (a) Give **one** sporting example of an open skill. Justify your answer. [3]
   (b) Which **one** of the following tennis skills is simplest? [1]
   - ☐ A – Hitting a forehand from a stationary practice position
   - ☐ B – Making a drop shot
   - ☐ C – Returning a serve
   - ☐ D – Striking a backhand volley in match play

   (c) Skills can be classified as being open or closed or anywhere in between.

   | Open skills | | | | Closed skills |

   Where on the environmental continuum above would you place a long jump?
   Indicate by placing an X on the continuum. [1]

3. Jo has started playing badminton with the hope of competing for her local club one day. Her instructor has provided a performance goal to help her improve her accuracy and to perfect specific movements in gameplay.

   Jo has committed a number of unforced errors (errors when she was in full control and not under pressure) and has set herself a target to achieve.

   Jo has collected the following data relating to her unforced errors in recent matches:

Match	1	2	3	Target
Unforced errors	39%	34%	30%	15%

   Table 1

   (a) Explain why the instructor has set a goal to help motivate Jo. [2]
   (b) Analyse the data in Table 1. Identify **two** ways in which Jo could better make her target goal meet the SMART principles. [2]
   (c) Explain **one** way in which goal setting can help to reduce injury. [2]
   (d) Jo is shown a video by her coach of a new technique to help improve her service returns.
   (i) State what type of guidance the coach is using. [1]
   (ii) Give **one** advantage and **one** disadvantage of this type of guidance. [2]

   OCR GCSE **Physical Education**

4. Using a sporting example, state how selective attention can increase the chances of successfully carrying out a skill for a performer. [2]

5. Knowledge of performance and knowledge of skills are types of feedback.
   (a) Which **one** of the following is an example of knowledge of results? [1]
      ☐ A – A cyclist being told their split times through sections of a race
      ☐ B – A discus thrower hearing a cheer from the crowd after their throw
      ☐ D – A gymnast instinctively knowing they 'nailed' a routine
      ☐ C – A skier being told to put more weight on the downhill ski
   (b) Discuss the use of knowledge of performance and knowledge of results for a beginner golfer. [4]

2.3

HEALTH, FITNESS AND WELL-BEING

Well-being means to be comfortable, healthy and happy. Health and fitness are related but they are not the same thing. Exercise plays a role in both.

Health

Health is defined as **a person's complete state of physical, mental and social well-being and not merely the absence of disease or infirmity**. All physiological systems need to be in positive, balanced harmony.

Decreased health may affect the intensity, regularity and desire to train or exercise, lowering fitness.

Fitness

Fitness describes **a person's ability to meet or cope the demands of their physical environment**. They should be able to physically perform an activity or task without increased risk of injury.

Fitness can still be increased despite poor health, for example if someone has an unhealthy diet, but is still able to train.

Mohammed said that "Abdi is healthy because he is not physically ill or frail".

(a) Explain what is incorrect about this statement. [2]

(b) Give **two** ways that health may be improved through greater fitness. [2]

(a) Abdi could have low self esteem / stress / depression / suffer from loneliness / poor posture / high blood pressure / alcohol or drug abuse / smoking habit / poor diet[1] which may not impact his physical condition / impacts his complete state of well-being.[1]

(b) Answers may include two from: Reduced chance of illness and disease / better sleep patterns / improved posture and personal image / stronger heart and reduced risk of heart disease / lower blood pressure / reduced risk of diabetes through reduced body fat / better social life if training together with others.

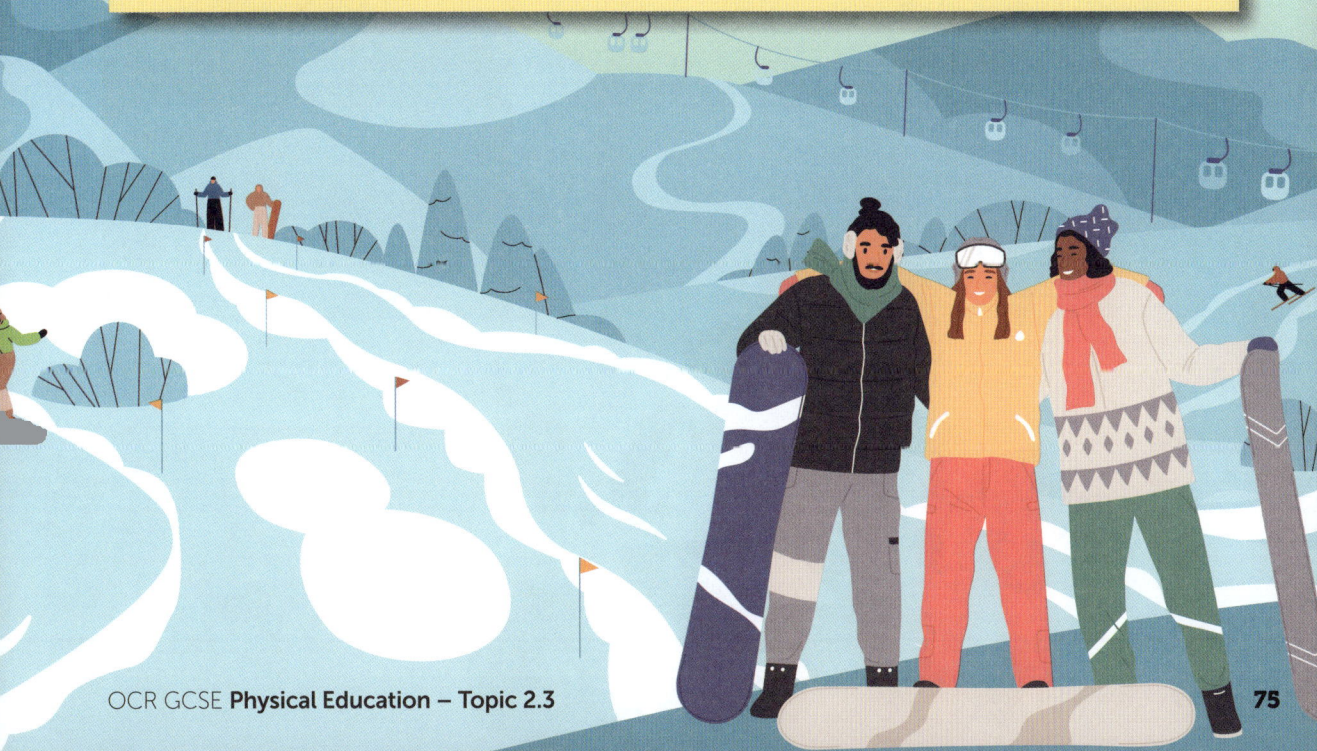

OCR GCSE **Physical Education** – Topic 2.3

THE HEALTH BENEFITS OF PHYSICAL ACTIVITY

Each component of **well-being** is positively impacted by participation in sporting activities. They form part of a set to keep you healthy with each element working in conjunction with the others.

Physical health and wellbeing

Physical health and wellbeing is defined as having all body systems working well, and being free from illness and injury with the ability to carry out everyday tasks.

Physical health:
- improves heart function
- improves the efficiency of the body systems
- reduces the risk of illness, e.g. diabetes
- means people are able to do everyday tasks without tiring
- helps to avoid obesity
- improves posture.

Social health and wellbeing

Social health and wellbeing mean that basic human needs are being met (for example, food, shelter and clothing). The individual has friendship and support, some value in society, is socially active and has little stress in social circumstances.

Social health:
- provides opportunities to socialise and make friends
- enables cooperation and teamwork
- ensures people have the essential human needs (food, shelter, clothing).

Emotional health and wellbeing

Emotional health and wellbeing is defined as how we think and feel about ourselves and others. This includes the ability to cope with life events, our own emotions and those of others in order to realise our own potential.

Emotional health:
- reduces stress, tension and anxiety
- helps with the release of feel good hormones (serotonin)
- increases confidence and self-esteem
- helps to alleviate depression
- helps people to control their emotions or anger.

BMI (**Body Mass Index**) is not on the specification, but it provides a rough approximation of obesity. Use the chart below to calculate your BMI.

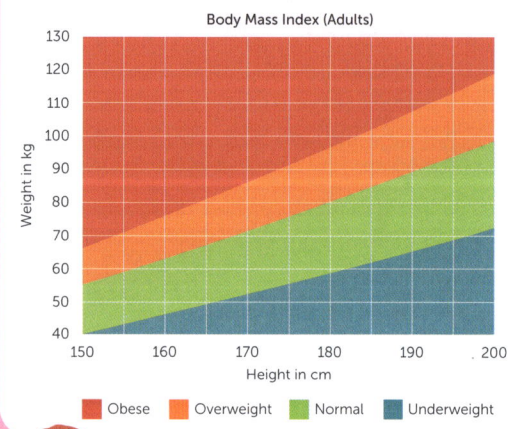

2.3

THE CONSEQUENCES OF A SEDENTARY LIFESTYLE

Our **lifestyle** is the way in which we choose to live. This includes our choices over what to consume, how often to exercise and our employment decisions. A **sedentary lifestyle** is one with irregular or no physical activity.

Consequences of a sedentary lifestyle

A sedentary lifestyle can involve spending long periods in front of the TV or sitting at a desk. Possible consequences of a sedentary lifestyle include:

Physical health
- Injury
- Coronory heart disease (CHD)
- Hypertension (high blood pressure)
- Decreased bone density
- Type 2 diabetes
- Poor posture
- Poor fitness
- Weight gain or obesity
- Heart disease
- Poor sleep

Emotional health
- Low self-esteem and confidence
- Poor stress management
- Self-conscious of image

Social health
- Friendships suffer
- Less opportunity to belong to a group
- Loneliness

> Explain **two** ways in which a sedentary lifestyle can impact physical health and wellbeing. [4]
>
> *A lack of exercise can result in consuming more calories than are burned through exercise,[1] leading to weight gain.[1] If the heart does not get exercise, it gets weaker and has to work harder / fatty deposits can build up in the arteries[1] leading to hypertension / heart disease.[1] A lack of exercise can cause muscle cells to lose their sensitivity to insulin,[1] causing diabetes.[1] Lack of resistance exercise can cause a drop in bone density[1] increasing the risk of fracture or osteoporosis.[1] Exercise helps to prevent insomnia / reduces stress[1] to improve sleep.[1] More likely to develop ill health,[1] lowering life expectancy.[1]*

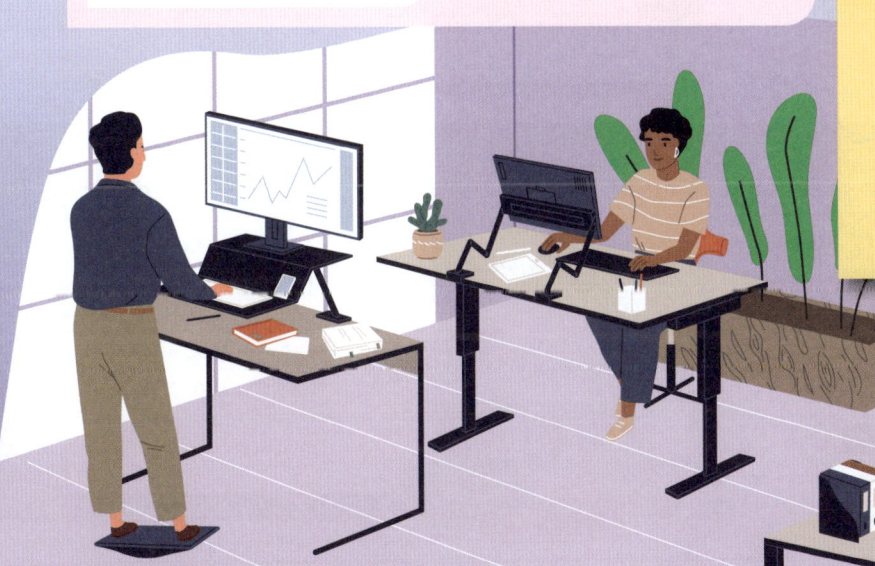

OCR GCSE **Physical Education** – Topic 2.3

2.3

BALANCED DIET

A **balanced diet** contains lots of different types of food to provide the right nutrients, vitamins and minerals required by your body.

A balanced diet

A balanced diet is defined as eating the right type and the right amount of nutrients that your body requires, consuming only as many calories as your body burns each day. Excess calories are stored as fat. A calorie deficit can cause a reduction of body mass through fat and muscle loss.

Increasing the amount of exercise you do, will require an increase in calories and nutrients, for example, additional protein to help muscle growth.

There is no single food that contains all the nutrients the body needs.

The reasons for a balanced diet

1. The body needs sufficient calorific energy available for its activity.
2. The body needs the correct nutrients for growth and hydration.
3. Consuming too much can create unused, or surplus, energy which is stored as fat. This could cause obesity (particularly with saturated fat).
4. To make sure that we get the right vitamins and minerals to prevent diseases such as rickets or scurvy.

Rickets is caused by a lack of vitamin D and calcium affecting bone development or weakening them in adults.

Scurvy is caused by a lack of vitamin C, causing tiredness, joint pain and bleeding gums.

Which **one** of the following meals provides the best balance of nutrients for a distance cyclist the day before a major competition? [1]

- A – Four cheese macaroni with sausage
- B – Bacon, lettuce and tomato sandwich
- C – Grilled chicken, leek and sweet potato pasta with broccoli
- D – Vegetable stir fry with rice

C.[1] (Balance of carbohydrates for energy, protein for muscle repair, rich in vitamins and minerals and low in fat.)

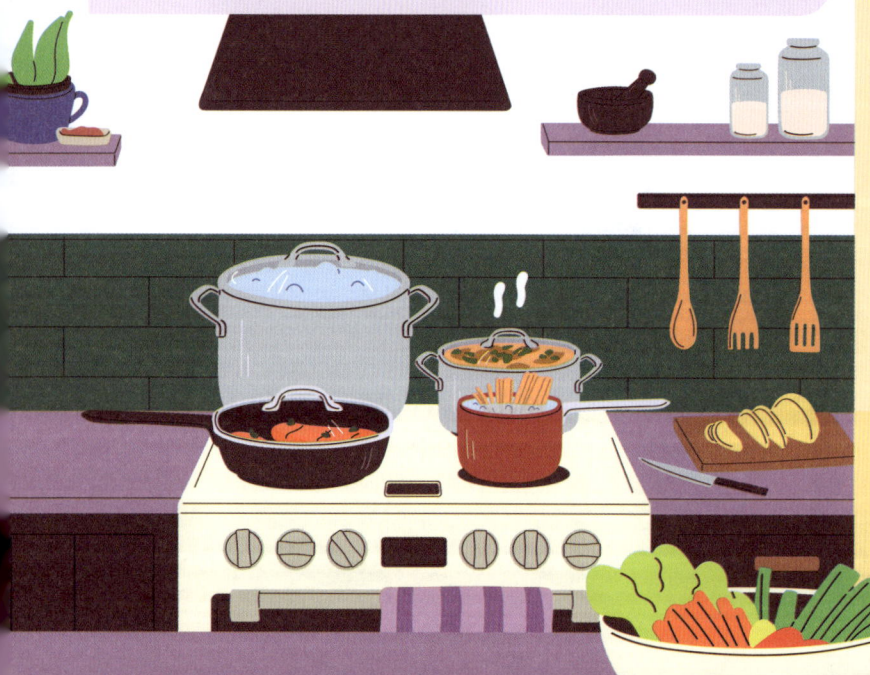

2.3

NUTRITION

Nutrition is defined as the intake of food, considered in relation to the body's dietary needs. Good nutrition is an adequate, well-balanced diet, combined with regular physical activity.

The role of carbohydrates, fat, protein and vitamins or minerals

A balanced diet contains roughly 55–60% carbohydrate, 25–30% fat and 15–20% protein. This can come from eating a variety of fruits and vegetables; bread, rice and pasta; meat, fish and eggs; and milk and dairy products. **Water** is also an important part of a healthy diet.

Carbohydrates

Carbohydrates (e.g. bread and pasta) are the main and preferred **energy** source for all types of exercise, of all intensities.

Protein

Protein is required for **growth and repair** of muscle tissue, developing strength.

Fat

Fats (e.g. oils and cheese) are essential for the body, though some types are better than others. Fat provides more **energy** than carbohydrates but only at low intensity, for example walking or jogging. Fat provides **insulation**, it protects vital organs with additional **cushioning** and supports **cell growth**.

Minerals

Minerals, such as calcium, are for **bone growth**, maintaining the efficient working of the body systems and for **general health**.

Fibre

Fibre (e.g. from grains and vegetables) **aids digestion**, **reduces cholesterol**, and limits obesity, diabetes and certain cancers.

You do not need to know about specific vitamins and minerals.

Vitamins

Vitamins (e.g. from fruit and vegetables) help to **prevent disease** and assist in the production of energy. They are essential for **metabolism** and aid tissue growth and repair.

---

1. Explain why a sprinter needs plenty of carbohydrates and protein in their diet. [4]
2. Give **one** health risk as a result of consuming more than the recommended 25–30% fat. [1]

1. Carbohydrates are burned at varying intensities, unlike fat, so their bodies can break down the carbohydrates into glucose for increased energy during intense training and competition.[1] Carbohydrates would therefore be the preferred energy source of the body.[1] Protein helps to develop muscular strength so they can increase their power and race times.[1] Outside training and competition, the muscles require protein to repair themselves.[1]

2. Heart disease,[1] high cholesterol,[1] hypertension (high blood pressure caused by a narrowing of the arteries).[1]

2.3

EFFECT OF HYDRATION ON ENERGY USE

People need to have enough water for the bodies to function normally. **Dehydration** refers to an excessive loss of body water, interrupting the function of the body. Rehydrating means to consume water to restore correct levels.

Consequences of dehydration

 Blood will thicken (increase in viscosity) with less water content, which slows blood flow, meaning less oxygen is supplied to the working muscles and to the brain. It also means that waste products such as CO_2 and lactic acid cannot be removed as efficiently.

 The heart will have to work harder, as a result of blood thickening, to supply oxygen to the working muscles during exercise. It may also develop an irregular rhythm. This could result in a poorer performance for a sports person.

 The body could increase in temperature (overheat) causing dizziness or fainting. This could prevent a performer from continuing their training or activity.

 Reaction times slow down as the brain is receiving less oxygen and muscles get tired. This can result in poor decision making and reduced skill levels.

 Muscles will tire, causing cramps, a limited range of movement and potentially preventing activity from continuing.

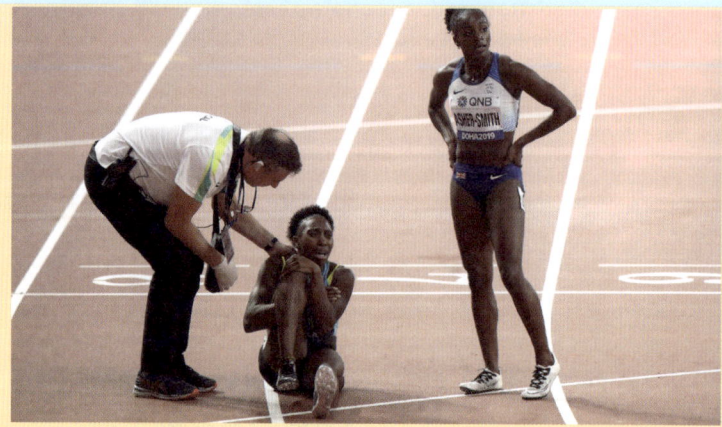

A sprinter of the Bahamas pulled up with cramp in the Women's 200m semi-final of the IAAF World Championships at The Khalifa International Stadium, Doha, Qatar.

(a) Give **one** cause of cramp. [1]

(b) Explain how the sprinter may have adjusted her water intake for the championships in the hot, dry climate in Qatar. [1]

(a) Dehydration / tired muscles / insufficient oxygen to the working muscles.[1]

(b) Increase water intake[1] in order to compensate for increased loss of water through sweating / increased evaporation in the breath.[1]

Topic 2.3

EXAMINATION PRACTICE

1. Which **one** of the following is a benefit of mental health and wellbeing? [1]
   - ☐ A – Improved heart function
   - ☐ B – More able to complete everyday tasks
   - ☐ C – Reduced risk of physical illness
   - ☐ D – Reduced stress

2. Participating in sports improves social health and wellbeing.
   - (a) Define social health and wellbeing. [1]
   - (b) State **two** positive effects that being physically active can have on social health and wellbeing. [2]
   - (c) Explain how better health could help improve fitness. [2]

3. Obesity can cause social, physical and mental ill health.
   - (a) Give **one** way in which obesity can negatively impact mental health. [1]
   - (b) State **one** way in which a person's body fat percentage can be reduced. [1]
   - (c) An adult has decided to reduce their BMI. Table 1 shows their progress over 6 months.

	Jan	Feb	Mar	Apr	May	Jun
BMI score	28	26	25	24	23.5	23

Table 1

Plot the BMI points onto the graph below and draw a line between them showing the trend. Label the axes. [2]

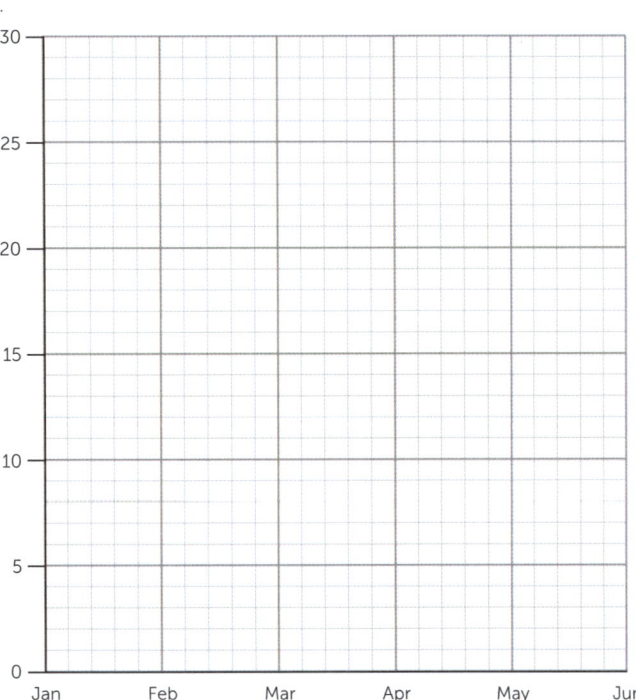

OCR GCSE **Physical Education**

4. Long distance cyclists in the Tour de France regularly consume water or liquids as they compete. Give **two** reasons why they need to hydrate. [2]

5. Protein helps with the growth and repair of muscles.
   (a) Which **one** of the following meals has a high protein content? [1]
      ☐ A – Leek and potato pie
      ☐ B – Grilled chicken with black beans
      ☐ C – Avocado salad with cucumber and mayonnaise
      ☐ D – Spinach and ricotta ravioli
   (b) Give **one** physical activity where a performer requires high levels of protein as part of their regular diet. [1]

6. Fibre and fat are essential to a balanced diet.
   (a) Give **one** reason for a balanced diet. [1]
   (b) Give **one** food source of fibre and **one** food source of fat. [2]
      Fibre: _____
      Fat: _____
   (c) Give **one** role of fibre and **one** role of fat in the body. [2]
      Fibre: _____
      Fat: _____

7. Is this statement true or false? Draw a circle around your answer. [1]
   A balance diet involves ensuring an equal proportion of fats, carbohydrates, vitamins, fibre and proteins in each meal.

   True

   False

8. There are social consequences of active and sedentary lifestyles.
   (a) Explain **one** social consequence of a sedentary lifestyle. [1]
   (b) Explain **one** social consequence of an active lifestyle. [1]

THE USE OF DATA

Specification coverage

The use of data analysis skills are spread across the components and topics.

Requirements

Demonstrate an understanding of how data are collected – both qualitative and quantitative

Present data, including graphs and tables.

Analyse and evaluate data, including graphs and tables.

UNDERSTANDING HOW DATA IS COLLECTED

The collection of data is crucial to analysis and the formation of conclusions. How data is collected often depends on the type of data that is required.

Quantitative data

Quantitative data is objective information which can be defined without opinion. It deals with numbers for example a score, distance, time or level. For this reason, it is more easily statistically analysed. Methods for collecting quantitative data commonly include **questionnaires** and **surveys**.

In a survey of 100 members of a local sports club, a questionnaire asked for the number of hours of exercise that respondents undertook each week. It also asked for their resting heart rate. Question 1 was segmented by hour to allow for easier analysis.

1. In the average week, how many hours of vigorous exercise do you complete?

| 0 | 1 | 2 | 3 | 4 | 5 | 6 | 7 | 8 | 9+ |

2. After a period of 20 mins after exercise, what is your resting heart rate in BPM?

64

Qualitative data

Qualitative data involves subjective information and deals with descriptions. This includes opinions and emotions. Interviews and observations allow for more detailed and descriptive responses.

Whilst conducting the same survey, interviews with some members collected the following response to exercise patterns:

"I love running on cold mornings, but I tend not to bother if it is raining."

Observations can be used to judge human behaviour over time to find patterns. The manager of the sports club observed that sports club members tended to change their use over time.

"A lot of people have high levels of exercise in January but that quickly tails off until the summer when longer evenings bring more people outside."

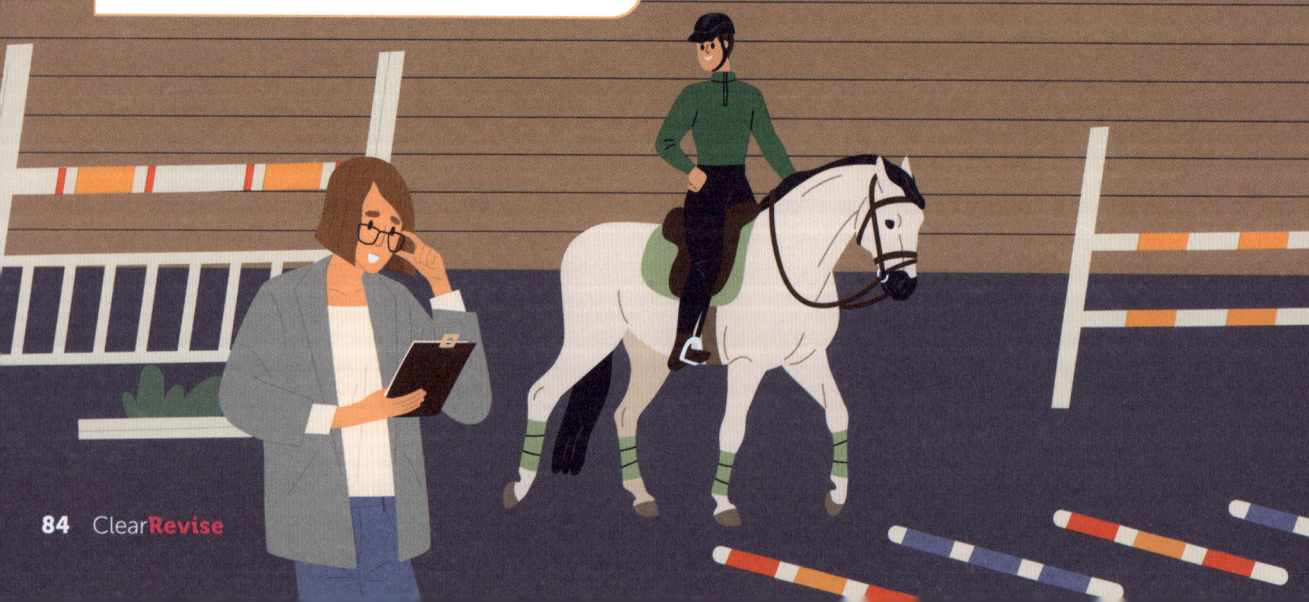

PRESENTING DATA

Data can be presented in graphical formats to show patterns more clearly.

Presenting data in tables

The data collected from the sports club survey can be tallied and averaged in a **table**:

Exercise hours per week	Frequency	Average resting heart rate
0	3	78
1	16	75
2	24	72
3	17	68
4	12	69
5	10	66
6	8	65
7	3	63
8	5	61
9	2	57

24 people exercised for 2 hours per week

Plotting basic bar charts and line graphs

Using the data in the table above, a **bar chart** (figure 1) can be plotted to show the number of people that exercise for 0–9 hours per week. A **line graph** (figure 2) can be plotted to show the average heart rate for club members for each level of exercise.

Figure 1: Bar chart

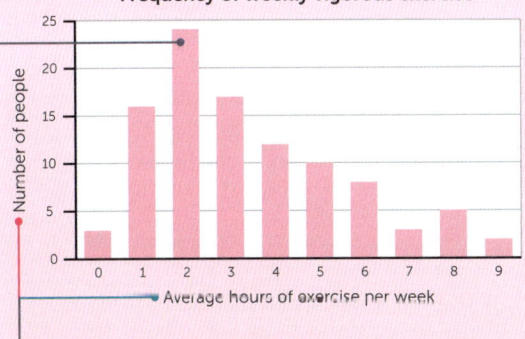

Figure 2: Line graph

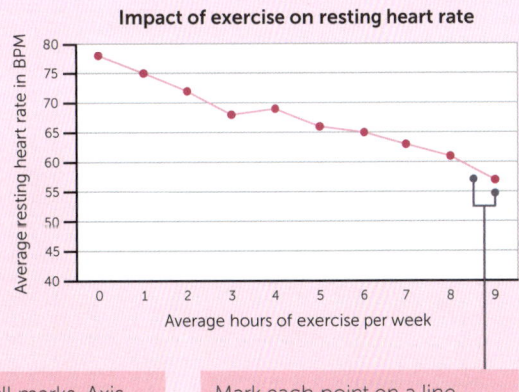

Always label the **x** and **y** axes on charts and graphs for full marks. Axis labels should include the units, for example: people, BPM or weeks.

Mark each point on a line graph, then join the markers.

Look at the line graph in Figure 2. Suggest the relationship between resting heart rate and hours of exercise in this sample of people. [1]

Those who did greater amounts of weekly exercise had lower resting heart rates. [1]

OCR GCSE **Physical Education** – The use of data

ANALYSIS AND EVALUATION OF DATA

Once data has been collected, it can be analysed, graphed and then interpreted. An evaluation of the data can more easily be made after this process.

Interpreting tabular data

The data in the table below shows the number of medals won by the GBR team in the Summer Olympics since 1992. Without some analysis, data tables can be difficult to interpret.

Medals	Barcelona 1992	Atlanta 1996	Sydney 2000	Athens 2004	Beijing 2008	London 2012	Rio 2016	Tokyo 2021
Gold	5	1	11	9	19	29	27	22
Silver	3	8	10	9	13	18	23	20
Bronze	12	6	7	12	19	18	17	22

This data could be analysed, for example, by sorting or by finding the totals for each year:

Total	20	15	28	30	51	65	67	64

Figure 1: GBR Summer Olympic medals since 1992

1. From the table of data presented in Figure 1, identify the most successful year for the GBR team in terms of gold medals won. [1]

   2012.[1]

Interpreting graphical data

Bar charts

Data presented graphically is often clearer and easier to extract useful information from.

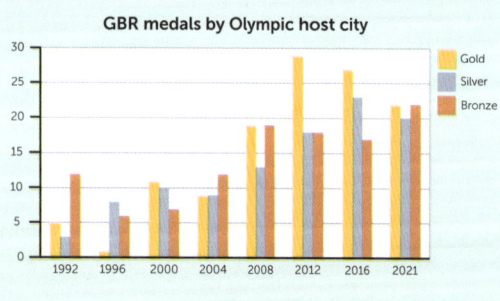

Figure 2

2. Look at the bar chart presented in Figure 2. Suggest **two** possible reasons why the performance of GBR athletes improved after 1996. [2]

   (National Lottery) funding was diverted into elite sport in 1996.[1] A new high-performance system spread across UK sports, putting the concept of marginal gains at the heart of training.[1] New, raw talent was better nurtured.[1] Team spirit increased in Beijing 2008 and the winning feeling has increased confidence and pride in athletes and their performance directors.[1]

Interpreting graphical data continued

Line graphs

Line graphs are often useful to see **trends** within the data. A trendline can also be added.

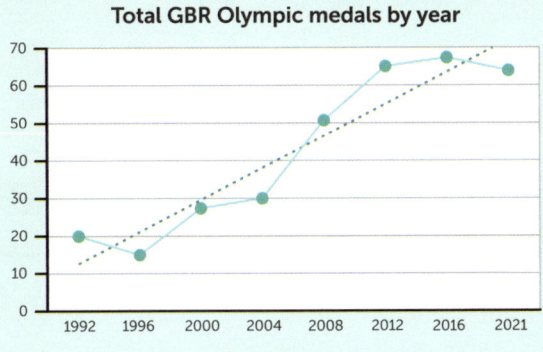

Figure 3

3. From the line graph presented in Figure 3, suggest the number of GBR medals likely in 2024.
Give a reason for your estimate. [2]

60–70[1] medals based on a plateau since 2012.[1] / 70–85[1] based on the trend line.[1]

Pie charts

Pie charts are used to show the proportions of a whole. In analysing charts, it is often helpful to look for **patterns**, **similarities** and **differences** by **comparing** sets of information. For example, two data points on a graph could be compared, or two points in time.

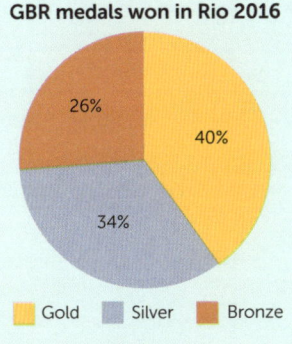

Figure 4

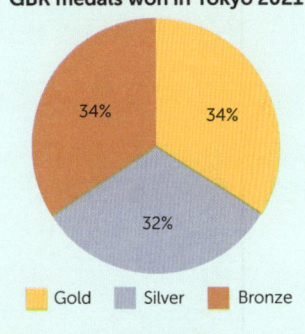

Figure 5

4. Look at Figures 4 and 5. Analyse the performance of the GBR team in both years. [2]

The proportion of silver medals remained at roughly a third.[1] Bronze medals increased in 2021 whilst gold medals decreased / potential gold or silver medallists may have lost out to gain a silver or bronze instead.[1] Performance was roughly consistent from one year to the next.[1]

 Make comparisons where possible and draw conclusions from data using the information provided and your own knowledge.

EXAMINATION PRACTICE

1. Which **one** of the following is an example of qualitative data? [1]
   - ☐ A – The Austrian skier has won five previous world champion slalom events
   - ☐ B – His split time was slower in the middle section by +0.42
   - ☐ C – The Austrian skier looks uncomfortable at the moment
   - ☐ D – He placed fourth in this race

2. Figure 1 shows a table containing the number of yellow cards handed out over six seasons for Windham Athletic football team.

Season	2017/18	2018/19	2019/20	2020/21	2021/22	2022/23
Yellow cards	58	71	49	44	42	41

   Figure 1

   (a) Draw a bar chart using the graph paper below and the data provided in Figure 1. [2]

   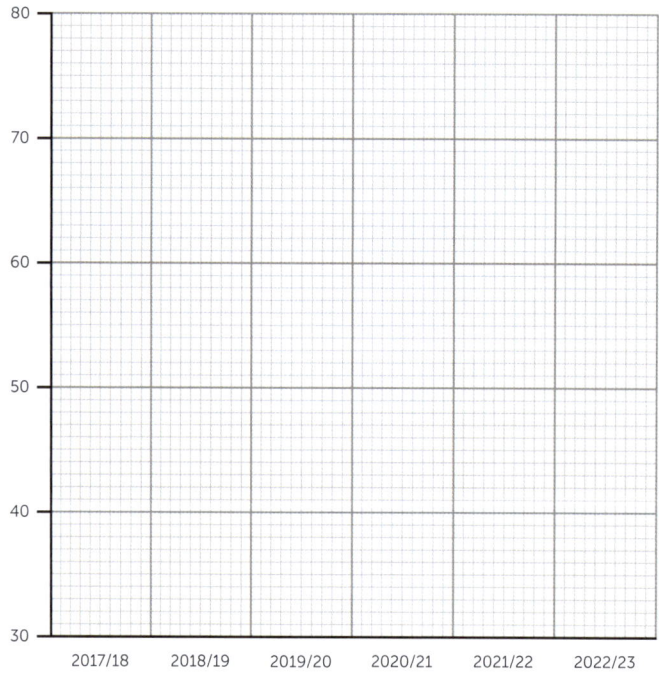

   Interpret the data in Figure 1.
   (b) Identify **one** piece of outlying or anomalous data from the series. [1]
   (c) Identify the trend shown in the data. [1]
   (d) Suggest **two** reasons for the trend. [2]
   (e) Suggest what the number of yellow cards is likely to be for the 2023/24 season. [1]

NON-EXAM ASSESSMENT (NEA)
Practical performance in physical activity and sport

Information about the non-examined assessment:

Assessed by teachers
80 marks
40% of the qualification grade

1. **Practical performances – 30% of the total GCSE: 60 marks**

   The three activities that you choose must come from the lists below and should include:
   - A team activity,
   - An individual activity, **and**
   - Any other activity of your choice

   Team sports:
   Acrobatic gymnastics, association football, badminton, basketball, camogie, cricket, dance, figure skating, futsal, Gaelic football, handball, hockey, hurling, ice hockey, inline roller hockey, lacrosse, netball, rowing, rugby league, rugby union, sailing, sculling, squash, table tennis, tennis, volleyball, water polo.

   Specialist sports: blind cricket, goalball, powerchair football, table cricket, wheelchair basketball, wheelchair rugby.

   Individual sports:
   Amateur boxing, athletics, badminton, canoeing / kayaking (slalom or sprint), cycling, dance, diving, equestrian, figure skating, golf, gymnastics, rock climbing, sailing, sculling, skiing, snowboarding, squash, swimming, table tennis, tennis, trampoline, windsurfing.

   Specialist sports: Boccia, polybat.

2. **Analysis and evaluation of performance – 10% of the total GCSE: 20 marks**

PRACTICAL PERFORMANCES

Your non-examined assessment requires you to take part in **three** different activities, evidencing specific skills and your performance in the full context of each sport.

Skills and decision making

Each of the activities have a list of **core skills** and **advanced skills** that should be performed, as well as demonstrating various **decision making** areas and elements of **tactical awareness**.

Sports performances will be recorded for evidence. For each, you should ideally:

- Aim to demonstrate improvement of performance.
- Demonstrate the full range of core, advanced and specific skills in isolation and under pressure in a competitive environment.
- Show tactical or compositional awareness during the performance.
- Demonstrate an understanding and application of the relevant rules, regulations and code of practice in the activity.
- Indicate the physical attributes of the performer, for example the level of physical fitness and psychological control demonstrated.
- Exhibit appropriate team strategies, tactics or compositional ideas to demonstrate an excellent understanding of the activity.
- Express excellent regard for the safety of themselves and others.
- Display excellent awareness of the strengths, weaknesses and actions of other players or performers in team sports.
- Show excellent communication with other players or performers in team sports.

Look at the relevant page in the specification for more detail about your chosen activity, for example, dance should be in front of an audience.

> **! Note**
>
> Evidence of activities that cannot be filmed at school, e.g. skiing or rock climbing, must be filmed and accompanied with detail such as the colour gradient of the piste or the difficulty rating of the climb.

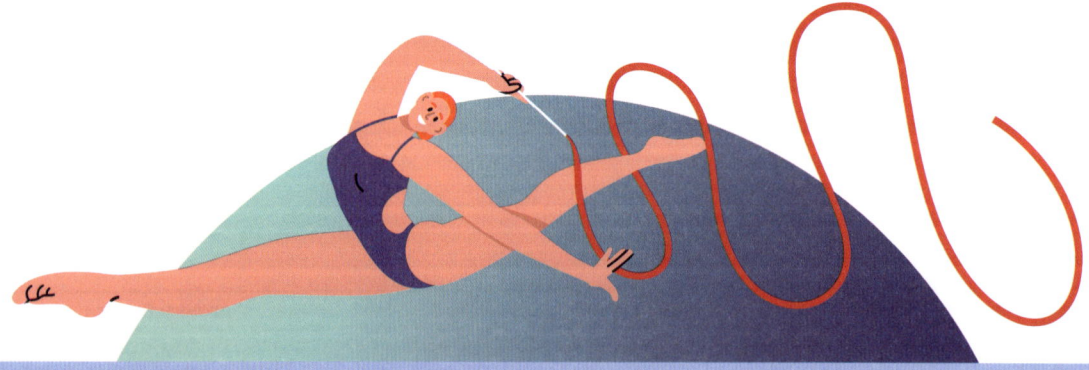

ANALYSIS AND EVALUATION OF PERFORMANCE (AEP)

You are required to demonstrate your ability to analyse and evaluate your own practical performance or that of a peer.

The AEP task

The AEP task needs to cover the following areas:

1. **Evaluation** of the physical fitness, strengths and weaknesses of the performer, relating them to the tests for each component of fitness.

2. **Analysis** of the relevance and importance of each component of fitness for the activity

3. **Overview** of all of the key skills required for your chosen activity.

4. **Assessment** of your own, or a peer's, strengths and weaknesses of the skills involved in the chosen activity.

5. **Movement analysis** of a joint, type of movement or muscle function, including the identification of where the movement sits on the appropriate continuum.

6. **Action plan** detailing how to improve an aspect of the performance such as a skills or component of fitness with relevant drills and practice. This should include a risk assessment, coaching points, application of SPOR And FITT, and SMART goal setting.

> Most students will type this section of their coursework. The action plan should be detailed but does not need to be physically carried out.

When completing this work, it is advised that you title each section to make it clear. For example, in the evaluation section, you are likely to title the following areas:

- Results of fitness tests
- Assessment and comparison of results to normative values
- Application to practical activity

> The fitness components and tests are listed on **pages 29 to 36** of this guide.
>
> The skills and techniques are listed in the specification under your chosen activity criteria.

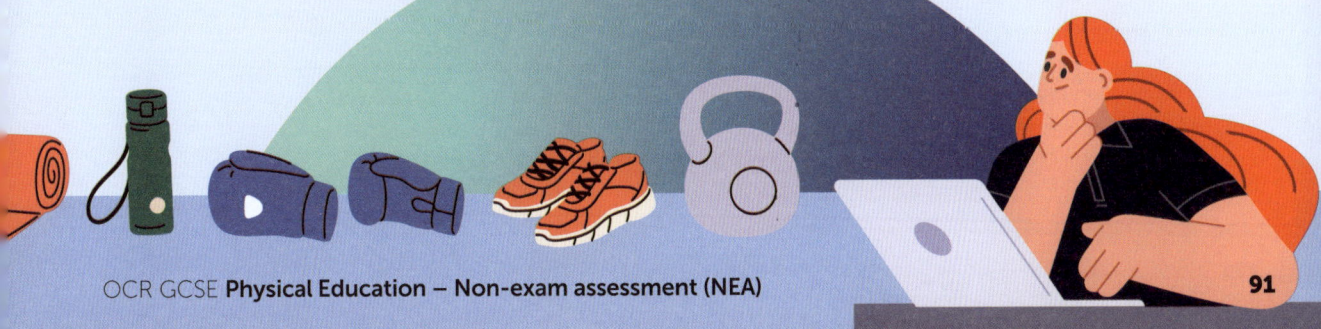

OCR GCSE **Physical Education** – Non-exam assessment (NEA)

EXAMINATION PRACTICE ANSWERS

Topic 1.1

1. A – Femur. [1]
2. True. [1]
3. (a) A – Left atrium → left ventricle → right atrium → right ventricle. [1]
   (b) Aorta carries blood away from the heart to the body. Vena cava carries it back again. [1] The aorta carries oxygenated blood. The vena cava carries deoxygenated blood. [1] The aorta transports blood from the left ventricle. The vena cava transports blood into the right atrium. [1] The aorta carries blood at high pressure. The vena cava carries blood at much lower pressure. [1] The aorta has thick walls to withstand the pressure. The vena cava has thin walls. [1] [4]
4. Support [1], protection of vital organs by flat bones [1], movement [1], to provide a structural shape [1], provide points for muscular attachment [1], for mineral storage [1] and blood cell production. [1] [3]
5. (a) Ligaments are less elastic than tendons. [1] Ligaments connect bone to bone / tendons connects bone to muscle. [1] Ligaments provide support and stability to a joint whereas tendons are designed to move the bone at a joint. [1] [2]
   (b) Provides a cushion for the joint in the event of impact.[1] Prevents bones from rubbing together / prevents wear and tear on the bones, causing pain.[1] [1]
6. (a) Tricep. [1]
   (b) The latissimus dorsi acts as a stabiliser[1] in the shoulder joint[1] to prevent unintended movement / to assist the agonists to work effectively.[1] [2]
7. (a) Third class / class 3 lever. [1]
   (b) Diagram must be labelled. Accept load/resistance. [1] [2]

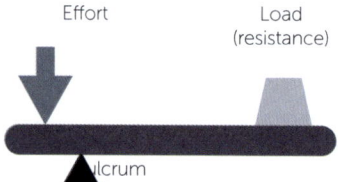

8. (a) (i) Plane – Sagittal. [1] Axis – Transverse. [1] [2]
       (ii) Plane – Transverse. [1] Axis – Longitudinal. [1] [2]
   (b) Extension. [1]
   (c) Effort arm is always shorter than resistance arm. / It has a short effort arm. / MA = effort arm / resistance (load). [1] Lever has low strength to effort ratio. [1] Lever is inefficient when considering strength. [1]

   3rd class levers allow a load to be moved more quickly / over a greater distance. [1] Third class levers always have an MA of less than 1. [1] [2]
   (d) Movement of the limbs (arms) away from the midline of the body. [1] Movement of the arms to the side [1] for balance. [1]
9. (a) C – Increased heart rate. [1]
   (b) This question should be marked in accordance with the levels-based mark scheme on **page 99**. [6]

   Indicative content may include:
   Knowledge of the effects on the body of long-term fitness e.g:

   Bone density, hypertrophy of muscle, muscular strength, muscular endurance, resistance to fatigue, hypertrophy of the heart, resting heart rate and resting stroke volume / lower resting heart rate (bradycardia), cardiac output increases, rate of recovery fastens, aerobic capacity increases, respiratory muscles strengthen, tidal volume and minute volume during exercise, capillarisation, body fat will be reduced over time.

   Application to an ice skater e.g:
   - Reducing body fat / weight / increased bone density will help with lifts, jumps and lessen the impact on landing.
   - Increased muscle mass / muscular strength in the legs will help with explosive power for jumps.
   - Suppleness and flexibility can help with the spin positions required.
   - Increased stamina can help a skater avoid fatigue before the end of their performance.

The importance of long-term fitness training to an ice skater e.g:
- Lifts and jumps are a core part of a skater's routine, so weight and strength need to be maintained.
- Performances can be improved through increased training, tailored to their needs so they maintain and increase their performance scores.
- A dip in fitness may result in a dip in performance scores so a faster rate of recovery would help with more regular training to maintain and improve fitness and skill levels.
- Variety is important to avoid boredom.
- They may need dietary supplements to increase carbohydrate intake which converts into glucose for energy, protein to help build and repair muscle (hypertrophy), fluids and salts for hydration and effective body function.
- SPOR and FITT need to be applied to ensure a safe and effective training program. Overload should be reached but not overdone.

10. Muscles are attached to bones by tendons. [1] When muscles contract, they pull on the tendon, which moves the bone. [1] Muscles work in antagonistic pairs. [1] As one contracts, the other relaxes. [1] Bones create lever systems which can be moved. [1] [3]

11. (a) Tidal volume shows the change in lung volume during a normal breath, in or out. [1]
    (b) It increases. [1]
    (c) Adrenaline may have caused it to increase. [1] A quick warm up on the side lines may have caused it to increase. [1] [1]
    (d) Intercostal muscles / sternocleidomastoid. [1]
    (e) The diaphragm contracts, moving downwards from a dome shape to a flatter shape. [1] The intercostal muscles contract moving the rib cage up and out. [1] This increases the volume inside the chest cavity. [1] Which decreases the pressure inside the chest cavity. [1] A pressure gradient is created, pulling air into the lungs through the nose or mouth. [1] [4]
    (f) Alveoli provide a large surface area for gas exchange to take place. [1] Walls are only one cell thick so gas molecules have a short distance to travel. [1] Oxygen moves from a higher concentration in the alveoli to the blood in the capillaries. [1] Carbon dioxide moves from the capillaries into the alveoli and into the lungs to be exhaled. [1] [3]
    (g) Can play basketball for longer / move body around the court more without getting tired. [1] Can play at a high intensity for longer without getting tired. [1] [1]

Topic 1.2

1. D – Decision making. [1]
2. B – Motor racing. [1]
3. A – Frequency. [1]
4. C – Cooper 12 minute run/walk test and the multi-stage fitness test. [1]
5. (a) Power is explosive strength / the product of strength x speed. [1]
   (b) Examples include: Sprinting to launch out of the blocks and sustain speed / hurdles / boxing to throw a fast, hard punch / shot put to launch the put / volleyball to spike. [1]
   (c) Standing vertical jump test. [1]
6. (a) Flexibility. [1] Increases muscular elasticity which reduces chance of injury / decreases muscle soreness. [1] Limbs have a greater range of movement so they can reach more shots / improve their technique. [1] Flexibility improves balance and mobility, keeping the player responsive / on their feet. [1]
   Cardiovascular endurance. [1] Increases the duration that they are able to perform at their peak with a raised heart rate. [1]
   Muscular endurance. [1] Avoids fatigue in muscles used repeatedly throughout a match. [1]
   Speed. [1] Helps a player to reach shots on the other side of the court / aids position between shots to return to the centre of the court. [1] [2]
   (b) Definition, 1 mark: The ability to move two or more body parts together smoothly and efficiently. [1]
   Importance, up to 2 marks: Hand eye coordination is required when hitting the ball. [1]
   The player must align their body with the incoming shot and position themself to strike with power. [1]
   The racket should hit the ball in the sweet spot so that they get maximum power on the ball. [1]
   To hit a ball on the move. [1]
   The player must move into the right position on the court to hit the ball before the ball reaches that point. [1]
   Better coordination should result in more shot points awarded / fewer unforced errors, competitive advantage. [1]
   A serve must be completed coordinated to throw the ball up and hit it perfectly. [1] [3]
7. David's score indicates that he has average agility. [1]
   Elizabeth's score indicates that she has good agility. [1]
   Even though David performed the test faster than Elizabeth, as a male, he is expected to be faster [1] / the scores compensate for males and females so Elizabeth is grouped in a higher performance category. [1] [3]

8. (a) Use the handgrip dynamometer in the dominant hand. [1] Squeeze the handle with maximum effort. [1] Keep the elbow at 90 degrees. [1] Keep the arm close to the body. [1] Record the best score. [1] [3]
   (b) This question should be marked in accordance with the levels-based mark scheme on page 99. [6]
   Indicative content may include:

   Knowledge of the grip test e.g:
   - The test measures grip strength.
   - The test does not measure the strength of any other muscle group.

   Application to a rock climber and a kayaker e.g:
   - A rock climber needs a strong hands and grip in order to hold on to a rock face.
   - A kayaker does not need a very strong grip, other than to hold onto the paddle.
   - The test is a standard test to measure grip strength with national benchmarks.

   The importance of the test to a rock climber and a kayaker e.g:
   - Grip strength is a fundamental skill for rock climbing as climbers need to use hand holds.
   - A kayaker needs to be able to hold on to the paddle, but there are far more important muscle groups such as the arms and back that depend more on strength in kayaking.
   - The test does, to some extent, replicate the movements of a rock climber using hand holds. It does not replicate the movements of kayaking.
   - Grip strength dynamometers may measure grip more in the whole hand rather than just the strength of the fingertips to cling onto a rock, so it may be limited as a measure of climbing ability.
   - Grip strength is a poor indicator of ability for a kayaker since it does not evaluate their overall strength, but it may provide some indication of general fitness and strength.
   - There are other standardised tests that may be better for both rock climbers and kayakers such as a sit-up bleep test or a wall toss test to measure muscular endurance and coordination.

9. FITT elements consider the frequency, intensity, time and type of training. Frequency can be increased gradually as fitness improves in order to increase stress on the body and increase overload. [1] Intensity measures how much stress is put on the body so as to see progression and put your body into the overload zone. [1] The time element considers the amount of time spent training which will need to be increased gradually with fitness levels to maintain overload and progression. The type of training helps with specificity so that the right training is prescribed for the right outcomes. [1] Type also helps alleviate boredom and potential reversibility as a variety of training methods can be used. [1] Type also ensures that training can work each of the different muscle groups to prevent overtraining and to balance overload. Type (variety) helps to maintain motivation, avoiding potential reversibility. [1] [3]

10. (a) Three from: Avoid over training [1], wear appropriate clothing and footwear [1], use PPE [1], compete at the appropriate level[1], use the correct technique [1], lift and carry equipment safely [1], cool down properly [1]. [3]
    (b) This question should be marked in accordance with the levels-based mark scheme on page 99. [6]
    Indicative content may include:

    Knowledge of plyometric training and other factors e.g.
    - Plyometric training involves jumping, bounding and hopping
    - It is good at developing power / explosive strength, but also speed
    - Training involves creating an eccentric contraction of a muscle which moves straight into a larger concentric contraction to maximise the length of the contraction and the power of the muscle movement
    - Diet may improve performance alongside any types of training
    - The principles of SPOR and FITT should be applied, regardless of the type of training
    - Callum should plan his warm-ups, rest periods and recovery.

    Application to Callum e.g.
    - Plyometric training can improve Callum's muscular endurance
    - Plyometric training can improve Callum's power
    - Plyometric training can improve Callum's speed
    - Power will be needed to avoid or quickly dodge an opponent
    - Callum will need a high level of fitness before starting plyometric training as it exerts high forces on muscles which could tear if he isn't already strong as there is a high risk of injury
    - If Callum adopts plyometric training during the football playing season, an injury could mean he misses the remaining fixtures
    - Callum would not need any specialist equipment and could practice plyometrics almost anywhere
    - He may need dietary supplements to increase his carbohydrate intake to convert this into glucose for energy, protein to help build and repair muscle (hypertrophy), fluids and salts for hydration and effective body function
    - SPOR and FITT need to be applied to ensure a safe and effective training program. Overload should be reached but not over done
    - Recovery practices should be put into place to reduce DOMS and prevent injury or tightness.

Evaluation of the appropriateness of plyometrics and other factors to Callum e.g.
- Plyometric training is well suited to improving speed and power in the legs which is a desirable attribute in a football player
- Football players needs speed when running for/with the ball so increased leg power will improve this fitness component for Callum
- Football players need explosive power in the legs to be able to respond to potential tackles, shoot or jump to head the ball so more powerful legs will help to improve the power and accuracy of a shot, improve height from a standing jump and improve the speed of response to avoid a tackle or fallen player.
- Training can be tailored to Callum to ensure that it is suitable for his current level of fitness and strength and that he has sufficient recovery time before the next match
- In a full match, other training methods may replicate the sporting movements of football more closely or provide greater benefits to Callum
- Callum could also combine plyometric training with other types of training to work on his cardiovascular (aerobic) endurance, core stability and agility such as interval training and circuit training to provide benefits of both aerobic and anaerobic exercise which reflects the stop/start nature of football and the bursts of energy required when a player prepares to get on the ball / gets the ball
- Ice baths, massages and a planned cool down routine including stretches will help reduce delayed onset muscle soreness (DOMS) and aid a faster recovery before the next match/training session
- Training should reflect the SPOR and FITT principles so that it is specific to Callum's needs, so that progress overload is reached and to avoid tedium.

Accept any other relevant points.

11. Warming up prepares your body for activity by raising heart rate / speeding up your cardiovascular system. [1]
Increased blood flow loosens the joints [1] and provides greater flow of oxygen to the muscles. [1]
Stretching prepares muscles for physical stress and improves the range of movement. [1] [2]

12. (i) Back pain and spinal injuries / dropped on foot. [1]
(ii) Scrum cap / helmet / shin pads / gloves / gum shield. [1]
(iii) Concussion / bruising / chafing / blisters / damage to teeth. [1]

Topic 2.1

1. It is summer, so provides a more appealing environment or climate to exercise outdoors in. [1]
2. Two from: disabled / less able [1], over 55s / older people [1], Asian / black / ethnic minority groups [1], lower socio-economic groups / lower income groups [1], minority faith groups [1], single parents.[1] [2]
3. (a) Lower the income, the higher the inactivity or the higher the income the higher the levels of activity. [1]
   (b) Award anywhere in the range 47% and 51% inclusive. [1]
   (c) 53.1 – 45 = 8.1% [1]
   (d) **Promotion:** [✓]
   Increase education [✓] by advertising the opportunities to get involved in sport / the health benefits / dangers of activity / inactivity. [✓] Increase media coverage [✓] in local newspapers and magazines of sports and minority groups involved in sports to encourage greater participation. [✓] Promote sport in schools for children under 16 [✓] to encourage more young people to get into a habit of a healthy lifestyle. [✓]

   Provision: [✓]
   Provide more facilities at county leisure centres / greater access to facilities [✓] through subsidised costs / bus services / extended opening hours (outside typical working hours). [✓] Provide childcare at gyms or sports clubs [✓] in order to provide a solution to parents who otherwise could not take part in activity. [✓]

   Access: [✓]
   Fund additional programmes for adapted sports [✓] to increase accessibility for disabled / less abled people. [✓] Create a (discounted) programme of sporting activities for the over 55 year old groups [✓] to increase the level of activity in these groups towards that of younger age groups. [✓] Introduce / subsidise more women's sports teams / events [✓] in order to boost participation by females. [✓]

   This question should be marked in accordance with the levels-based mark scheme on **page 99**. [6]

4. A – Commercialisation. [1]
5. (a) Money, [1] performers, [1] publicity, [1] increase. [1] [4]
   (b) One from: financial, [1] footwear, [1] nutritional support, [1] (e.g. Lucozade), scientific support (e.g. Rolex timing). [1] [1]

(c) Facilities e.g. stadia: The Etihad stadium at Arsenal / The Etihad Stadium at Manchester City. [1] Clothing: Umbro sponsor the sports kit for the England rugby team. [1] Equipment: Dunlop Slazenger supply all balls to Wimbledon. [1] Accept any other examples. [2]

6. Any two named media types with explanation. Television [1] can be live or via a highlights programme [1]. Radio [1] can be free to air such as BBC 5 live [1]. Social media [1] accounts can be updated 24/7 to provide information, facts and opinions [1]. Internet [1]. Fan and club websites can update the public on all matters relating to the sports club [1]. [4]

7. Max 2 marks as the third match is determined by the first two. [2]

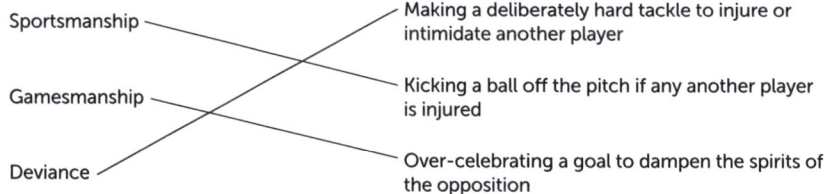

8. (a) True. [1]
   (b) A – Anabolic steroids. [1]
   (c) Two from: Improve concentration [1], suppress fatigue [1], releases protected reserves of energy [1], raise confidence levels [1], increase aggression. [1] [2]
   (d) The reputation of boxing and boxers could be heavily damaged. [1] People may lose trust in past and future results. [1] The sports body could lose their key sponsorship leading to a loss of income. [1] Spectator numbers and the overall fan base may reduce, reducing interest, media coverage and income from ticketing and merchandise. [1] Participation levels may fall if grass roots performers perceive that success is only possible with performance enhancing drugs. [1] There would need to be a difficult, awkward and embarrassing process to revisit previous results so that belts and titles could be redistributed to fair performers. [1] More funding would need to be invested into drug testing instead of helping emerging or elite athletes to perform to higher standards. [1] Honest or 'clean' athletes can lose credibility if they are suspected or assumed to drug users. [1] [4]

9. Instinctive response, [1] e.g. hitting back / pushing. [1] Pressure to win, [1] e.g. hindering the performance of others / intimidation through violence. [1] Nature of the game, [1] as contact (or close contact) sports are more likely to incur outbreaks of violence e.g. high rugby tackle / elbow in football. [1] Frustration of losing or being penalised, [1] can cause a backlash against the opposition or officials. [1] Retaliation / intimidation, [1] to hard tackle another player as a result of an earlier tackle / to keep them quiet for the match. [1] Copying others with poor form or attitudes, [1] can result in doing the same again to others. [1] [2]

Topic 2.2

1. Predetermined skills include: gymnastics routine / high dive / figure skating routine / penalty kick / javelin throw. [1]
   Aesthetic skills include: Bent football shot / slam dunk / snowboard air / gymnastics aerial. [1] [2]

2. (a) Sailing. [1] The environment is constantly changing (wind / current / waves) which the performer needs to make adjustments for. [1] The performer needs to respond to movements by opponent boats in order to outwit them / make counter movements. [1] Movements are performed differently depending on which direction the boat is facing / aiming to go. [1] [3]
   (b) A – Hitting a forehand from a stationary practice position. [1]
   (c) Accept anywhere in the 'closed' half. [1]

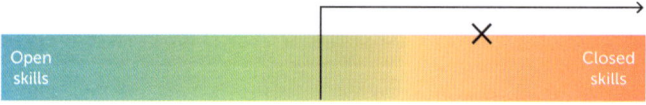

3. (a) As a beginner, Jo could be demotivated by unrealistic targets. [1] Jo may be more likely to train if there are specific goals to achieve. [1] Jo may not be motivated to be the best at this stage, just to be the best she can be. [1] Jo needs to focus on her own skills rather than those of others to improve. [1] Goals may help Jo to optimise her performance. [1] Her own performance goals cannot be affected by others, so they are more likely to be achieved by a beginner. [1] [2]
   (b) Recorded – Jo needs to log all her forced and unforced errors in order to calculate her percentage. [1]
   Achievable – 15% may be too low / difficult to achieve depending on the time frame she has to achieve this. [1]
   Timed – Provide a definitive date by which she must achieve the target. [1] [2]
   (c) Achievable goals / goals agreed with a coach / realistic goals [1] are less likely to push performers beyond their maximum causing mental or physical stress. [1] Measurable / recorded goals may provide challenge which motivates performers to use the correct (safe) technique / warm up and cool down properly. [1] [2]

(d) (i) Visual guidance. [1]
   (ii) Allow error carried forward from part (i).
   Advantages: Quick, concise which is especially good for beginners so they can copy. / Slow motion replays (pausing) can be used for detailed analysis of complex skills. / Can see what to do and form a model of the movement. [1]
   Disadvantages: Complex skills can be difficult to demonstrate clearly. / Performers need to be paying close attention. / Harder to 'feel' the movement or understand the process. [1] [2]

4. Award max one mark for a suitable example and one mark for description. A footballer taking a direct free kick [1] can use selective attention to block out distractions from the crowd / the opposition [1] which increases their focus / concentration on taking the free kick. [1] [2]

5. (a) A – A cyclist being told their split times through sections of a race. [1]
   (b) Response must relate to the context. A beginner golfer would benefit from knowing how they have performed as it provides advice and reassurance / allows them to improve their swing / putting. [1] Knowing their results provides a concrete target to improve on [1] but they may be discouraged by relatively poor results in the round / hole. [1] Knowledge of results immediately after each shot / hole is helpful as quick feedback on which to build [1] however, knowledge of the score for the whole round or over a series of rounds can take time and be more frustrating to wait for. [1] Knowledge of results concentrates on the outcome [1] whereas knowledge of performance focuses on the technique used to achieve an outcome. [1] The golfer may 'feel' when they have made a good or bad shot before the ball lands through their own intrinsic knowledge of performance. [1] Knowledge of performance tends. [4]

Topic 2.3

1. D – Reduced stress. [1]

2. (a) Basic human needs are being met (food, shelter and clothing). The individual has friendship and support, some value in society, is socially active and has little stress in social circumstances. [1]
   (b) Two from: Opportunities to socialise with other people, [1] make friends, [1] enjoy some teamwork or team sports, [1] / cooperate with other people. [1] [2]
   (c) Improved mental health / self-esteem / appearance / reduced depression [1] could improve the desire to train or exercise (in public). [1] Improved blood pressure / diet / quitting smoking [1] could make exercise easier to approach / more enjoyable / more manageable. [1] Improved friendship groups / social standing / reduced loneliness [1] may provide greater desire / opportunities to train socially. [1] [2]

3. (a) One from: Depression, [1] loss of confidence, [1], anxiety, [1] stress. [1] [1]
   (b) One from: Consume fewer calories. [1] Increase energy expenditure. [1] [1]
   (c) Award one mark for points correctly plotted on the graph. One for correctly labelled axes. [2]

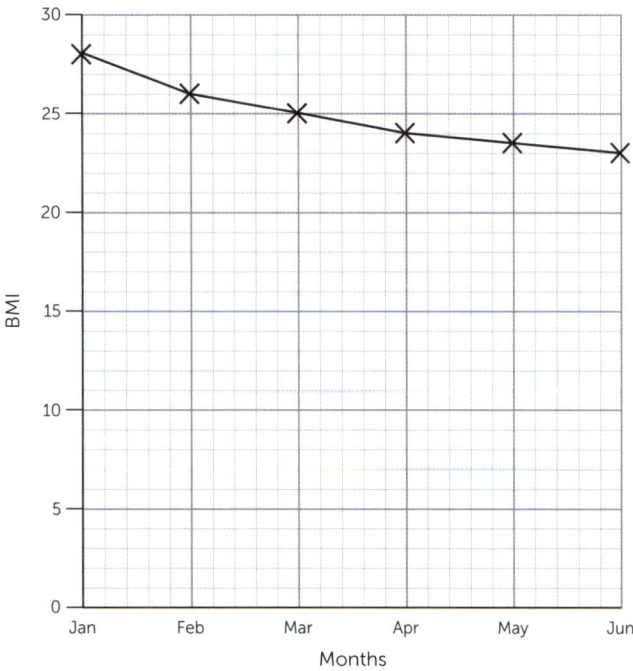

4. To replace fluids lost through sweat or increased evaporation in the breath. [1] To regulate body temperature / reduce heat exhaustion. [1] Reduce the chance of tiredness / fatigue in the working muscles. [1] To quench their thirst. [1] [2]

5. (a) B – Grilled chicken with black beans. [1]
   (b) Example of a physical activity where power and explosive strength are required. E.g. boxer, weight lifter, sprinter, sprint swimmer. [1]

6. (a) One from: Unused energy is stored as fat, which could cause obesity, [1] suitable energy can be available for activity, [1] the body needs nutrients for energy, growth and hydration. [1] [1]
   (b) One from: Fibre – Fruit / vegetables / wholemeal cereals / brown rice / beans / nuts / seeds.
   One from: Fat – Vegetable oils / nuts or seeds (if not given for fibre) / fish / dairy produce. [2]
   (c) Fibre aids digestion / helps to reduce cholesterol / reduces the risk of disease (diabetes) / helps maintain a healthy weight (limits obesity). [1] Fats provide reserve energy / insulation / protection of the vital organs / support for cell growth. [1] [2]

7. False. [1]

8. (a) One from: Friendships may suffer [1] as they may all partake in physical activity / may stop inviting you out to join them / which can lead to loneliness. [1] Lose the feeling of belonging to a group / club [1] which can lead to loneliness. [1] [1]
   (b) One from: Becoming more active may take away from social time outside sports [1] which may reduce contact with friends [1] Acceptance from within an active group of friends may alienate other groups who are less active [1] as a result of envy / difference of opinion / rejection. [1]

The use of data

1. C – The Austrian skier looks uncomfortable at the moment. [1]
2. (a) Correctly labelled x axis (Season/Year) and correctly labelled y axis (Number of yellow cards). [1] Bars correctly plotted for each season. [1] [2]

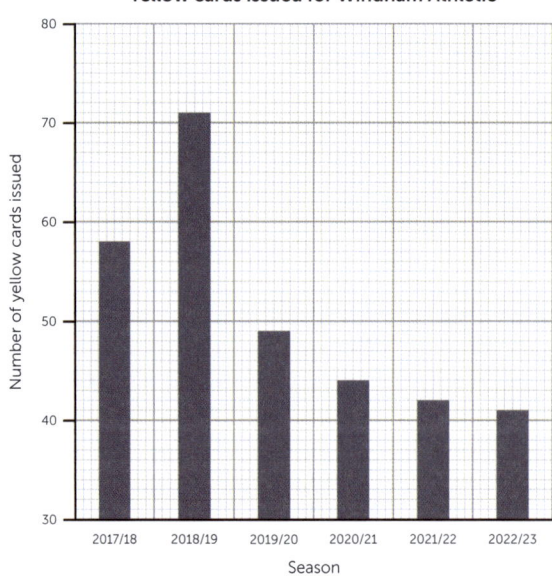

   (b) Data for 2018/19 (71) was much higher than other data points and outside of the trend. [1]
   (c) Yellow cards generally decreased over the six year period. [1]
   (d) Two from: Change of manager with stricter policies on foul play. [1] Change in FA regulations. [1] Club incentives for players to reduce bookings. [1] Change in referee(s). [1] Change in playing style and technique. [1] Greater fitness / ability of players. [1] Greater team bonding and morale. [1] Accept any other reasonable response. [2]
   (e) Accept between 38 and 41. [1]

LEVELS-BASED MARK SCHEME FOR EXTENDED RESPONSE QUESTIONS

What are extended response questions?

Extended response questions are worth 6 marks. These questions are likely to have command words such as 'compare', 'explain' or 'evaluate'. You need to write in continuous **prose** when you answers one of these questions. This means you must write in full sentences (rather than in bullet points), organised into paragraphs if necessary.

You may need to bring together skills, knowledge and understanding from two or more areas of the specification. To gain full marks, your answer needs to be logically organised, with ideas linked to give a sustained line of reasoning.

Some extended response questions may involve calculations. These need two or more steps that must be done in the right order. These questions are likely to include the command word 'calculate'.

Marking

Calculations are **not** marked using 'levels of response' mark schemes, but longer written answers are marked this way.

Examiners look for relevant points (indicative content) but they also use a best fit approach. This is based on your answer's overall quality and its fit to the descriptors for each level.

Example level descriptors

Level descriptors vary, depending on the question being asked. Level 3 is the highest level and Level 1 is the lowest level. No marks are awarded for an answer with no relevant content. The table gives examples of the typical features that examiners are asked to look for.

Level	Marks	Level descriptors
3	5–6	• Response contains detailed knowledge and understanding. Comments are relevant to the context of the question. • Responses are always clear, showing correct application of knowledge to the context of the question. Several relevant points, views, or opinions may be presented. • Effective analysis, discussion and development of relevant points, drawing on other relevant areas of the specification. • Comparisons and contrasts may be discussed. • Accurate use of technical terms and specialist vocabulary. • A clear and well-developed line of reasoning has been demonstrated.
2	3–4	• Response contains satisfactory knowledge and understanding relating to the question. • Some responses correctly apply knowledge and reasoning to the context of the question. • Some relevant information referenced in the development of a response but there will be limited analysis of any relevant factors related to the question. • More than one relevant response will have been included. • Technical terms used with some accuracy. • A line of reasoning with some structure has been demonstrated.
1	1–2	• Basic knowledge and understanding. • Responses rarely apply any knowledge to the context of the question. • Little or no reference to other information or attempt to develop a point. • Limited use of or relevance of technical terms. • Responses are unstructured and supported by limited evidence.

INDEX

Symbols
1 Repetition Maximum (1RM) test 32
30m sprint test 31

A
abdominal muscles 8, 19
abduction 6
ability 67
access 55
adduction 6
advertising 58
aerobic exercise 21
aesthetic skill 66
age 51
agility 31
agonist 9
alveoli 18
anabolic steroids 62
anaerobic exercise 21
ankle 2
antagonist 9
aorta 16
arteries 14, 16
artificial outdoor areas 46
Astroturf 46
atria 14
axes of rotation 13

B
balance 34
ball and socket joints 5, 6
bar charts 85, 86
beta blockers 62
biceps 8, 32
blood
 cells 4, 15
 flow 45, 80
 lactate 23
 pooling 44
 vessels 16
BMI (Body Mass Index) 76
bones 2, 79
 density 24
 marrow 4
BPM (beats per minute) 17
bradycardia 24

brand image 58
breathing 19
breathing rate 20, 45
bronchi 18
bronchioles 18

C
calcium 4, 78
calories 78
capillaries 16, 18
capillarisation 24
carbohydrates 79
cardiac output 17, 22, 24
cardiovascular endurance 29
carpals 3
cartilage 5
chambers 14
cholesterol 79
circuit training 40
circumduction 7
clavicle 3
closed skill 67
clothing 45
collar bone 3
commercialisation 56
competition 45
complex skill 67
components of fitness 29
continuous training 38
continuum 66, 67
cool down 44, 45
Cooper 12 minute run/walk test 29
coordination 35, 66
cranium 2
culture 53

D
data 84, 85
deltoid 8
deviance 60
diaphragm 19
diet 78
difficulty continuum 67
diffusion 16, 18
disability 54
discrimination 51, 52, 53, 54

donations 58
double circulatory system 14
drugs 62
dynamic movements 43

E
education 51, 54
efficiency 66
effort 10
elbow 3
elbows 5, 6
emotional health 76, 77
energy 21, 79
environmental continuum 67
equipment safety 45
ethics 60
ethnicity 53
exercise
 long-term effects 24
 short-term effects 22
exhalation 19
expiration 19
explosive strength 33, 41
extension 6
extrinsic feedback 72

F
fair play 60
family 54
fartlek training 39
fat 4, 78, 79
fatigue 24, 80
feedback 72
femur 2, 3
fibre 79
fibula 3
fine skills 66
fingers 3
first class lever 10, 12
fitness 29, 75
fitness centres 46
FITT 37
fixator muscle 9
flexibility 33
flexion 6
fluency 66
footwear 45

frontal axis 13
frontal plane 13
fulcrum 10

G

gamesmanship 60
gas exchange 14, 16, 18
gastrocnemius 8
gender 52
glucose 21
gluteals 8
goal setting 68
golden triangle 56
graphical data 86
grip strength dynamometer test 32
gross skills 66
guidance 70

H

haemoglobin 18
hamstrings 8
hazards 46
head 2
health 75
health benefits 76
heart 14
heart rate 17, 22, 44
high intensity interval training 42
hinge joints 5, 6
hip flexors 8
hips 5, 6
humerus 2, 3
hydration 80
hypertrophy 24

I

Illinois agility test 31
imagery 69
inhalation 19
injury prevention 45
inspiration 19
intercostal muscles 19
internet 57
interval training 40
intrinsic feedback 72

J

joints 4, 5, 6

K

kinaesthetic feedback 72
knee 3, 5, 6
knee cap 3
knowledge of performance 72
knowledge of results 72

L

lactic acid 21, 23, 44, 45
latissimus dorsi 8, 32
levers 4
lever systems 10
ligaments 5
line graphs 85, 87
load 10
longitudinal axis 13
lumen 16
lungs 18

M

magazines 57
manual guidance 71
marrow 4
mechanical advantage 12
mechanical guidance 71
media 56, 57
media coverage 51, 52, 54, 55
mental rehearsal 69
merchandising 58
metabolism 79
metacarpals 3
metatarsals 2
minerals 4, 78, 79
minute ventilation 20, 23
minute volume 24
mobility 43
motor skills 66
movement 4, 6, 9
multi-stage fitness test 29
muscles 4, 8, 9, 23
muscular continuum 66
muscular endurance 24, 30, 41
musculoskeletal system 2

N

negative feedback 72
newspapers 57
nutrition 79

O

open skill 67
organs 4
osteoporosis 24
overload 37
oxyhaemoglobin 18

P

participation 55
participation in physical activity 51
patella 3
pathway of air 18
pectoral muscles 19
pectorals 8, 32
pelvis 2
performance enhancing drugs 62
personal protective equipment 45
phalanges 3
phosphorus 4
physical activity 50, 76
physical health 76, 77
pie charts 87
planes of movement 13
playing field 46
plyometric training 41
positive feedback 72
positive thinking 69
power 33
pre-determined movements 66
press-up test 30
prime mover 9
principles of training 37
progression 37
promotion 55
protein 79
provision 55
pulmonary loop 14
pulse raising 43

Q

quadriceps 32
quadriceps group 8
qualitative data 84
quantitative data 84
questionnaires 84

R

radius 3
reaction time 36, 80
red blood cells 15
rehearsal 69
religion 53
resistance 10
respiratory
   muscles 19, 24
   rate 20, 23
   system 18
retaliation 61
reversibility 37
rib cage 19
ribs 2
role models 52, 53, 54, 55
rotation 7
ruler test 36

S

sagittal plane 13
scapula 3
second class lever 11, 12
sedentary lifestyle 77
selective attention 69
self-talk 69
shoulders 3, 5
simple skill 67
sit and reach test 33
sit-up Test 30
skeleton 2, 4
skilful movement 66
skill rehearsal 43
skills classification 67
SMART targets 68
social
   grouping 51
   health 76, 77
   media 57
specificity 37
speed 31
spine 2
spirometer 20
sponsorship 56, 58
SPOR 37
sport 56
   in the UK 50
sports halls 46
sportsmanship 60
stamina 29
sternocleidomastoid 19
sternum 2, 3
stimulants 62
stork stand test 34
strength 32, 41
stretching 43
stroke volume 17, 22, 24
surveys 84
swimming pool 46
synovial joint 5
systemic loop 14

T

tabular data 85, 86
tarsals 2
tendons 5, 8
third class lever 11, 12
tibia 3
tidal volume 20, 23, 24
toes 3
trachea 18
training 38, 45
transverse axis 13
transverse plane 13
trapezius 8
triceps 8
TV and visual media 57

U

ulna 3

V

valves 14
vascular shunting 22
vasoconstriction 22
vasodilation 22
veins 14, 16
ventricles 14
verbal guidance 70
vertebrae 2
vertical jump test 33
violence 61
visual guidance 70
visualisation 69
vitamins 78, 79

W

wall throw test 35
warm up 43, 45
water 79
weight training 41
well-being 75, 76
working muscles 23
work:rest ratio 40

ACKNOWLEDGEMENTS

The questions in the ClearRevise textbook are the sole responsibility of the authors and have neither been provided nor approved by the examination board.

Every effort has been made to trace and acknowledge ownership of copyright. The publishers will be happy to make any future amendments with copyright owners that it has not been possible to contact. The publisher would like to thank the following companies and individuals who granted permission for the use of their images and extracts in this textbook.

All graphics and images not mentioned below © Shutterstock
Longjumper © Stefan Holm / Shutterstock.com
Basketball game © Pavel Shchegolev / Shutterstock.com
Pommel horse routine © Michele Morrone / Shutterstock.com
Throw-in © katatonia82 / Shutterstock.com
Long jump take-off © John Bingham / Alamy Stock Photo
Kayak sprint © Celso Pupo / Shutterstock.com
Pattaya Tadtong © FocusDzign / Shutterstock.com
Emma Lamb © Action Foto Sport / Alamy Stock Photo
Comber leisure centre © Ballygally View Images / Shutterstock.com
Novak Djokovic © Leonard Zhukovsky / Shutterstock.com
Mo Farah © Matthew Pull / Shutterstock.com
Emma Lamb, England Women's Cricket © Action Foto Sport / Alamy Stock Photo
England Men's Rugby © Marco Iacobucci Epp / Shutterstock.com
Etihad Stadium © 4kclips / Shutterstock.com
David Beckham © PA Images / Alamy Stock Photo
Tonya Harding © PA Images / Alamy Stock Photo
F1 press conference © GP Library Limited / Alamy Stock Photo
Angel Valodia Matos © Associated Press / Alamy Stock Photo
Evander Holyfield © Associated Press / Alamy Stock Photo
Taylor / da Silva tackle © PA Images / Alamy Stock Photo
Marion Jones © Allstar Picture Library / Alamy Stock Photo
Kim Jong-Su © dpa picture alliance archive / Alamy Stock Photo
Adrian Mutu © ph.FAB / Shutterstock.com
Matthieu Voisin © Mai Groves / Shutterstock.com
European Swimming Championship © Paolo Bona / Shutterstock.com
Taison Barcellos Freda © Oleksandr Osipov / Shutterstock.com
Nafissatou Thiam © SPP Sport Press Photo. / Alamy Stock Photo
AJ MacGinty © Action Plus Sports Images / Alamy Stock Photo
With thanks to Sport England for the use of their data.

NOTES, DOODLES AND EXAM DATES

Doodles

Key dates

Paper 1:

....

Paper 2:

....

EXAMINATION TIPS

When you practice examination questions, work out your approximate grade using the following table. This table has been produced using a rounded average of past examination series for this GCSE. Be aware that boundaries vary by a few percentage points either side of those shown.

Grade	9	8	7	6	5	4	3	2	1	0
Boundary	78%	73%	69%	64%	58%	52%	38%	25%	12%	0%

1. Read questions carefully. This includes any information such as tables, diagrams and graphs.
2. Remember to cross out any work that you do not want to be marked.
3. Answer the question that is there, rather than the one you think should be there. In particular, make sure that your answer matches the command word in the question. For example, you need to recall something accurately in a **describe** question but not say why it happens. However, you do need to say why something happens in an **explain** question.
4. Use connective words in your answers, for example, 'because', 'such as', or 'so that' as these force you to give an explanation for your answer, commonly gaining an additional mark in questions worth two or more marks.
5. Ensure that your responses have the appropriate amount of depth based on the number of marks provided and avoid repeating the same point in a variety of ways.
6. Ensure any sporting examples are relevant to the context of the question.
7. In longer answer questions involving levels of response, be sure to include AO1 (knowledge and understanding), AO2 (application of knowledge) and AO3 (analysis and / or evaluation). Give detailed reasons and focus on the impact in AO3. These questions also commonly include knowledge from both sections of the theory specification.
8. Both the examination papers will include multiple-choice questions (MCQs). Make sure you neatly tick the answer you want to be marked. If you change your mind, put a cross in the box (from corner to corner). If you change your mind back again, put a circle neatly around the box.
9. Show all the relevant working out in calculations. If you go wrong somewhere, you may still be awarded some marks if the working out is there. It is also much easier to check your answers if you can see your working out. Remember to give units when asked to do so.
10. Plot the points on graphs accurately and use a ruler. Ensure that you are drawing the type of graph asked for in the questions. Do not confuse bar charts with line graphs. Label all lever diagrams, graphs and charts fully.
11. Write legibly! Candidates often lose marks where examiners are unable to read their handwriting.
12. Write your answers on the lines provided. The lines are usually a good indicator of the length of the expected answer. If you need more space, use additional paper to complete this, clearly numbering the response with the question number. Make it clear that you have used extra paper in the answer space provided.

Good luck!

New titles coming soon!

These guides are everything you need to ace your exams and beam with pride. Each topic is laid out in a beautifully illustrated format that is clear, approachable and as concise and simple as possible.

They have been expertly compiled and edited by subject specialists, highly experienced examiners, industry professionals and a good dollop of scientific research into what makes revision most effective. Past examination questions are essential to good preparation, improving understanding and confidence.

- Hundreds of marks worth of examination style questions
- Answers provided for all questions within the books
- Illustrated topics to improve memory and recall
- Specification references for every topic
- Examination tips and techniques
- Free Python solutions pack (CS Only)

Absolute clarity is the aim.

Explore the series and add to your collection at **www.clearrevise.com**

Available from all good book shops

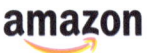 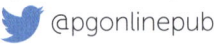 @pgonlinepub

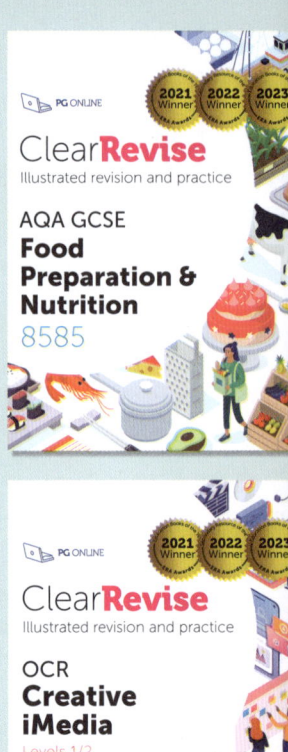

ClearRevise
Illustrated revision and practice
AQA GCSE
Food Preparation & Nutrition
8585

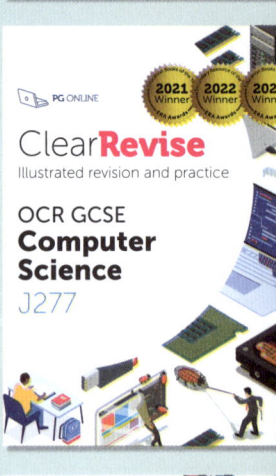

ClearRevise
Illustrated revision and practice
OCR
Creative iMedia
Levels 1/2
J834 (R093, R094)

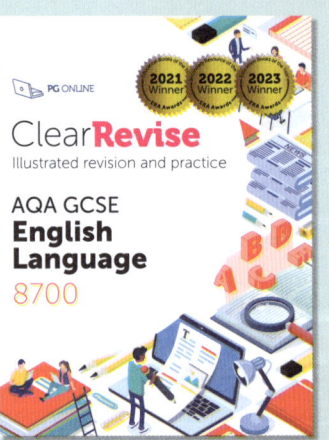

ClearRevise
Illustrated revision and practice
AQA GCSE
English Language
8700

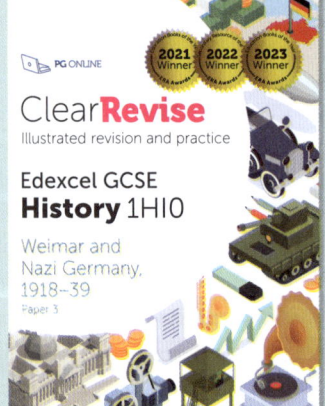

ClearRevise
Illustrated revision and practice
Edexcel GCSE
History 1HI0
Weimar and Nazi Germany, 1918–39
Paper 3

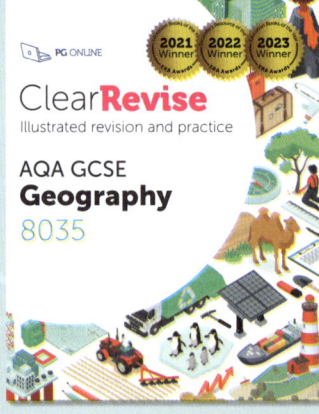

ClearRevise
Illustrated revision and practice
AQA GCSE
Geography
8035

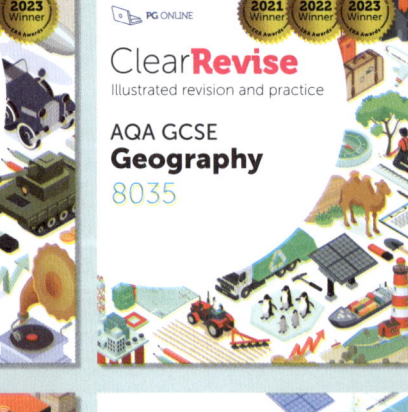

ClearRevise
Illustrated revision and practice
OCR GCSE
Computer Science
J277

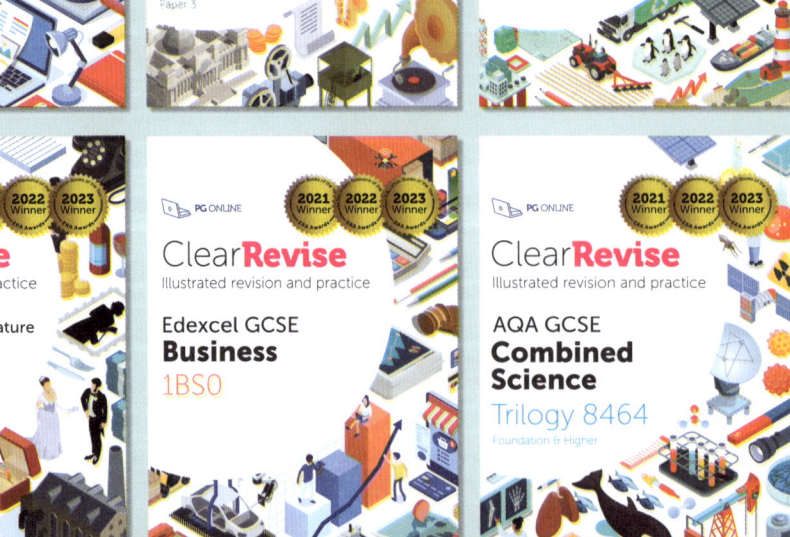

ClearRevise
Illustrated revision and practice
AQA GCSE English Literature
An Inspector Calls
By J. B. Priestley
8702

ClearRevise
Illustrated revision and practice
Edexcel GCSE
Business
1BS0

ClearRevise
Illustrated revision and practice
AQA GCSE
Combined Science
Trilogy 8464
Foundation & Higher

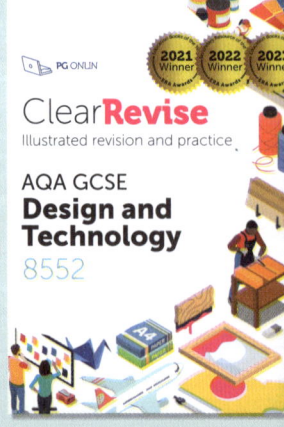

ClearRevise
Illustrated revision and practice
AQA GCSE
Design and Technology
8552